FemTruth™ Endometriosis Edition

A Collection of Stories by Courageous Women

By Silvia Young

Foreword by Heather Guidone

Cover Art by Jaimee Rae and Lleon Pascal

Prologue

I invited the endometriosis community to send in their stories. At the time, I thought I would individually edit and publish these on my Medium publishing platform. After reading them, I realized the strength of storytelling in women's circles, and a book blossomed.

The courage it takes survivors to revisit trauma and share it publicly for the greater good, is a testament to each other's perseverance and integrity. Putting grief and abuse into words is a humbling journey in and of itself.

But that's how warriors are made.

Sharing these stories, I hope other women find validation and inspiration. The Endometriosis life is a social injustice. Together, by sharing our experiences, we can find our truth and build a more just future for the next generation.

This book marks a celebration of empowerment for all our authors. Although cathartic, it's a huge journey to navigate and self-realize. A special thank you to all our readers too. Even reading these stories is breaking taboo and an act of rebellion.

Each story is a snapshot in time from 2018 of women dealing with a cruel and misunderstood disease estimated to impact "1 in 10" women.

A living document to bear witness to the Human Rights violations and the battle for justice.

Dedicated to endosisters all over the world.

Our Women's Circle is everything.

United by our FemTruth™

Table of Contents

FOREWORD	Heather Guidone, New York
ONE	Amy Jane Melhuish
TWO	Allenia Owens
THREE	Stephanie Parido
FOUR	Renee Papesh
FIVE	Joy Grey
SIX	Alyssa Sanchez
SEVEN	Anna Gaboury
EIGHT	Casey Berna, MSW
NINE	Stephanie Saure
TEN	Katrina Alleyne
ELEVEN	Silja Steinunnardottir
TWELVE	Samantha Bowick
THIRTEEN	Dr. Sallie Sarrel PT ATC DPT

FOURTEEN	Lisa Howard
FIFTEEN	Tricia Connelly
SIXTEEN	Cicely Daniels
SEVENTEEN	Nancy Peterson, RN
EIGHTEEN	Brandi La Perle
NINETEEN	Stephany Adeyemi
TWENTY/ TWENTY ONE	Jaimee Rae McCormack Laura Mccormack-Long
TWENTY TWO	Imogene McClain
TWENTY THREE	Dr. Wendy Bingham, DPT
TWENTY FOUR	Silvia Young

"It troubles me greatly that our children – and even grandchildren – are largely still struggling with the same diagnostic delays and poor treatment pathways I was subjected to decades ago."

– Heather Guidone

FOREWORD

Heather Guidone, New York

Thirty years ...

Thirty years is a long time. Over the span of three decades, medicine and technology have made incredible advances. Scientific breakthroughs have happened. Innovations have transformed our world, changing the way we think, work, teach, shop, learn and interact. New discoveries have improved – even revolutionized - our lives. Perhaps no field has emerged more in terms of growth and development than healthcare. From next-generation therapies to complex data assimilation, the face of medicine has grown by leaps and bounds, improving – and saving – lives every day.

Why then, the question begs, is endometriosis still stymied by the status quo and mired in virtually the same quagmire I fought through when I began my own personal (and a few years later, professional) journey with the disease in the late 1980s?

As a woman who has experienced Stage IV endometriosis, 'frozen pelvis,' adenomyosis, leiomyoma and primary infertility, it troubles me greatly that our children – and even grandchildren – are largely still struggling with the same diagnostic delays and poor treatment pathways I was subjected to decades ago. Where are the scientific advances in endometriosis, one may ask. Why, as Professor Sun-Wei Guo correctly terms it, does 'innovation drought' persist in this disease?

Having been professionally immersed in the patient care, research, education and advocacy sectors for more than two decades, I'm honored to have had the opportunity to be both student and teacher in the tireless fight to increase endometriosis awareness, expand the fundamental pathways towards better diagnosis and management, and achieve better policies in this disease. However, despite the best efforts of the incredible champions and thought leaders I have had the privilege of toiling beside, those who have truly moved mountains in the disease, one point is clear: we still have so far to go and there is much work left to be done.

Endometriosis exacts a vast and painful toll on lives, including my own: significantly reduced quality of life, compromised academic and professional opportunities, impaired sexual and physical functionality, negative effects on relationships, losses in productivity, "in your head" diagnoses that can lead to crippling self-doubt, hopelessness and isolation, countless ineffective medical and surgical treatments and more.

In a word: despair.

Those who do not live with endometriosis - while sympathetic - can never fully comprehend the perspective of pain, devastation, isolation and missed opportunities that are part and parcel of this disease.

Clinically speaking, endometriosis is the existence of endometrial-like tissue located in the extra-uterine environment. The disease commonly develops on pelvic structures like the ovaries, gastrointestinal tract, urinary tract and soft tissues, but is also routinely found outside the abdominopelvic region. Though similar, endometriotic lesions are molecularly distinct entities compared with eutopic endometrium. Simply put: it is tissue somewhat resembling, but not the same as, endometrium found outside the womb, elsewhere in the body where it doesn't belong.

The disease elicits a sustained inflammatory response, accompanied by angiogenesis, adhesions, fibrosis, scarring and neuronal infiltration, and there may be marked distortion of pelvic anatomy, development of painful endometriomas, and a high association with a number of comorbidities.

Endometriosis is also commonly associated with infertility, and compared to individuals without endometriosis, those with the condition have a worse health-related quality of life overall.

Wide-ranging symptoms of this heterogeneous disease may be systemic and become chronic over time. Though classically referred to as a 'disease of women,' endometriosis can impact all bodies; menstruators and non-menstruators alike, including rare cis males and trans-identified, gender non-conforming individuals. Nevertheless, the condition continues to be strongly linked to 'painful periods,' despite symptoms routinely impacting sufferers far and apart from menses.

Endometriosis affects an estimated 176 million individuals globally, at a staggering, annual fiscal tab to society soaring into the billions.

What these cold, clinical facts can't illustrate about endometriosis is that unless you have first-hand experience with a chronic, painful disease, one cannot truly imagine what it is like to be at constant war with your own body. My journey with endometriosis began early on – indeed, symptoms I could later identify and associate with the condition began even before my first period. Struggling with self-doubt, as so many with endometriosis do, I assumed my pain and symptoms were 'normal' - or maybe it was all in my head.

These messages were reinforced after finally seeking help, when doctors repeatedly told me I just needed to relax; I was 'stressed' and 'thought about my symptoms too much'. Best I should just take the sedatives they gave me and go about my business. When the medications didn't work, I blamed myself. My naïveté buttressed the patriarchal dynamics of those doctor-patient relationships; surely they knew far better than I - they were worldly physicians and I was merely a girl who was too high-strung with too low of a pain tolerance. I became complicit in my own mistreatment.

At a time that should have been the most socially formative and academically engaging, I was struggling in isolation with a silent enigma that would ultimately shape every aspect of my life. Analogous to living under the rule of a dark entity, it was endometriosis that decided every aspect of my life for many years. When I could go to work, engage in social pursuits and other activities, embark on travels – or even just leave the house on any given day. It was endometriosis that held command over the most intimate aspects of my relationship; sex was not a choice of my own doing. It was endometriosis that controlled whether, when or if having a child was an option.

Those around me were as tired of hearing "excuses" for not being present as I was of making them. Pain became a constant shadow; plans were made to be broken; goals were to be put on hold.

Then, in the late 1980s, one of the many physicians on my medical merry-go-round finally believed me. He told me my symptoms were real and "it might be endometriosis" – a word I had never heard of, didn't understand, and was ill-prepared for the implications of.

He suggested surgery to confirm the diagnosis; I agreed. A 9-hour, hip-to-hip open laparotomy later, I was validated: stage 4 endometriosis. That validation did not come without a price, however.

The surgeon delivered the most devastating news at my post-op bedside: I probably wasn't going to get any better, would never have children and needed to schedule a hysterectomy as soon as possible. I wasn't even of legal drinking age yet – but was suddenly faced with making choices about the rest of my life before the anesthesia had even worn off. Somewhere within my befuddled soul I found the resolve to decline his offer to 'cure me' by taking out my uterus. His second option? More medication and a therapist.

So life went on. As many who struggle with endometriosis do, I overcompensated. I didn't want to be 'that girl.' My career track was defined by long hours, high stress and near-impossible standards, but I did well and even thrived – if you don't count the fact that most days I wanted to crawl under my desk from pain and lay on the office floor sobbing, all while still smiling on the outside.

I became a master secret keeper, hiding my pain from everyone around me. I self-medicated. I nuanced the art of internalizing my pain. I wrote missives in private about my struggles (one of which, the Letter from Survivors, eventually found the light of day and made its way to more than a million readers around the globe), while publicly pretending nothing was wrong. At the end of most days, I had no energy left for anything else in life.

On 'good' days, I was bound and determined to be a part of the scene and keep up appearances, even to the detriment of my own health. My disease remained a secret I revealed only to a select few – for years. It is difficult to put into words the shame, fear, frustration, emotional, physical and financial consequences of this disease, even now.

The endeavor to get well was the constant backdrop to my life. Like having a second job, doctor's appointments, infertility counseling, new medications, old medications, repeated surgeries, alternative therapies and fending off well-intentioned but failed advice from those around me was an ever-present undertaking. I was exhausted simply from living.

There was no white picket fence and happy family with 2.0 children and a puppy. There was, however, a new husband who learned quickly that he had married both me AND my disease, feeling helpless while his wife was crippled by pain day after day. There were friends and family who didn't understand - and didn't care to ask. Travel? Go out to dinner? Sex? Not a chance. Vacations? Time away from work was reserved for sick days and surgeries. My best friend's wedding? Missed. I still hurt for these losses decades later.

In a serendipitous twist of fate, by the time I was at the lowest point in my health, I had segued into working in endometriosis full-time. I was also actively volunteering for disease efforts when I could and being an engaged activist to the extent my well-being would allow. I had access to "the best" doctors, the "most current" research, the most "forward-looking" therapies – or so I thought.

I trusted the countless physicians who told me they were doing all they could for me. I believed them when they said the incomplete surgeries they performed over and over on me, leaving disease behind, were the best that medicine could offer for my disease.

I took them at their word when they injected me with Lupron - 24 times - and cried behind closed doors when the side effects proved worse than the disease, some of which I still suffer from today, decades later.

I diligently swallowed the innumerable oral contraceptive formulations given to me, a cruel paradox for someone suffering from infertility.

I gave $600-per-hour Park Avenue "celebrity gyns" the benefit of the doubt when they insisted that hysterectomy had been the right suggestion early on. I blindly accepted their avowals that "there was no hope" for my case. After all, everything I had researched, everyone I spoke to, all the disease conferences I attended had established that these were indeed the correct protocols for endometriosis.

I was taught that living with the condition meant a lifetime of repeated interventions, no matter how poorly they failed me. This was the modus operandi of the disease, I was told, and I'd better learn very quickly to adapt to my New Normal.

But then, an epiphany, delivered by an endometriosis nurse 3,000 miles away. There was hope, and there was a better way. I could stay bitter, or I could get better. I chose the latter.

Years of pain, over twenty surgeries and countless drug therapies later, I finally met the doctor – himself located 1,000 miles away - who changed everything. The painstaking, six-hour excision procedure my surgeon – an actual endometriosis expert – and his team performed on my bowels, ureters, kidney, bladder, diaphragm, tubes, gall bladder, ovaries and cul-de-sac saved my life in ways only someone who has made it to the other side of this disease can understand.

As it turned out, I didn't have a low pain threshold after all – in fact, my medical team marveled at how "well" I had been persevering with the amount of damage I had suffered at the hands of clearly obvious disease. They didn't understand that, in fact, I was merely existing and everything else to the contrary was just smoke and mirrors, a pretense I had mastered to an art form.

My relief was short-lived, however – so I believed. About a month post-op, I became very ill. Blood work revealed a most shocking development: I was pregnant. At that moment, I knew I had overcome the worst endometriosis will ever throw at me.

To say my pregnancy was not easy is an understatement. I was confronted with some of the obstetrical risks endometriosis imposes, among the most serious being pre-eclampsia. I was managed very closely by a high risk obstetrician, treated for hyperemesis gravidarum, put on a Holter monitor, treated for gestational diabetes, monitored closely for miscarriage and other risks. I spent a great deal of time going in and out of the hospital and to specialist appointments, and was frightened often.

Ultimately placed on bed rest for my and the baby's well-being, I found myself undergoing an emergency induction six weeks early. My foray into motherhood began with a postpartum hemorrhage that necessitated yet another gynecologic surgery.

And yet, I would do it all again without hesitation. My son is perfect and just celebrated his 20th birthday as of this writing.

As I learned first-hand thirty years ago, the biggest barrier to effective care for the 176 million individuals struggling with the disease is still a lack of awareness at even the highest echelons of society. Stemming from a deep-rooted silence on menstruation and pelvic health in general which continues to pervade our culture - with pelvic pain particularly enshrouded by myths and misinformation, the lack of conversation contributes to the lengthy delays in diagnosis and poor treatment of endometriosis.

This incredibly symptomatic illness, which can lead to systemic pain, infertility and significantly altered lives, isn't talked about in polite company. We don't discuss painful periods, pelvic pain, bowel or urinary symptoms and other endometriosis-related affects over dinner, leaving many to suffer in silence.

Telling patients their pain is 'normal' further compounds the issues surrounding the disease. As a result, quality of care for endometriosis remains fragmented, with high treatment failures and consequent recurrence posing formidable challenges.

Despite its vast prevalence, diagnostic delays persist, globally averaging a decade before diagnosis is confirmed. Definitive cause remains elusive, as is universal cure or prevention, and much of the discourse surrounding etiology and treatments is ardently debated.

Unrelenting bias enshrouds menstruation and pelvic pain, keeping endometriosis often belittled, ignored, under-diagnosed, medicalized, inadequately treated and marginalized. Patients frequently feel isolated, and those suffering from associated menstrual pain may be disparaged as 'menstrual moaners' who are simply unable to cope with "typical period pain."

Unfortunately, both patients and doctors may still normalize symptoms of dysmenorrhea, rely on hormonal suppression therapy and inappropriately look towards nondiscriminatory investigations for diagnosis, further confounding the physical, emotional and social toll on the affected.

Rather than be attributed merely to a 'female's plight in life,' pelvic pain and/or severe dysmenorrhea that affects daily living and does not respond to medical intervention requires professional attention and must be given a proper diagnosis for underlying cause(s) e.g. endometriosis. Often, the disease is also sidetracked by a narrow-minded focus on fertility issues - when what healthcare providers should be focusing on is not an individual's procreative potential, but the impact pain has on that person's ability to make and enjoy their own choices; sexual, career or socially oriented.

Doctors and other healthcare professionals must engage patients in conversations which remain sensitive to cultural context, perceptions and attitudes, yet draw out possible symptoms and menstrual issues at first sign so individuals are treated in timely and effective ways that harmonize with their specific needs. Hysterectomy, drug therapy and ineffective surgery remain the routine recommendations, even today in our age of supposed medical advances and despite the fact that better options exist.

Gender bias continues to reign supreme in every aspects of women's health from research to treatment. Likewise, lack of disease education continues to be a significant barrier, and the shortage of accurate information about endometriosis across the public is staggering.

Continued propagation of myths and misconceptions by the media, practitioners, academia and patients alike persist, despite best efforts by many to promote modern concepts. The media constantly reports inaccuracies and promotes old myths about endometriosis; doctors still don't believe their patients; healthcare professionals still don't fully understand the disease; society still does not know about endometriosis; and many in our underfunded research community promote outdated notions in perpetuity.

It has been nearly a century since Sampson taught that endometriosis is normal endometrium in abnormal locations, developed through abnormal backflow (retrograde menstruation). Given our elevated knowledge now, we know that isn't the whole story - endometriosis and eutopic endometrium are histologically and biochemically different on a profound level, and many other flaws exist with Sampson's Theory, which does not explain pathogenesis in all patients, particularly in extrapelvic disease, men and other non-menstruators.

Unfortunately, these teachings still guide much of the treatment and research to this day. Endometriosis remains a highly politicized disease, where profits are often put over patients by the very organizations which shape the educational, treatment and funding protocols that the rest of us must live with. The institutional neglect of an entire system, which fails to recognize the specialty treatment of the disease, continues to prevent access to quality care.

That system isn't broken - they built it that way.

The outdated myths and misinformation about endometriosis, to say nothing of the bias and industry control over much of the research community, are a large part of the reason why more significant progress hasn't been made.

This must end.

We can't always control what happens to us in life, but we can control how we react to it and the person we become because of it. So, use your voice and tell your story. Remember that education is the key to making informed decisions about your care, and educating those around you will ensure that you have allies along your journey. When we know better, we do better; those struggling with endometriosis can only benefit from educating themselves as thoroughly as possible about all aspects of the disease utilizing trusted, credible sources.

Prepare for your next appointment by writing down important health information including medications, current symptoms and questions; keep track of and organize your medical information so you can be an empowered patient in your own care. Remember that you are the leader of your treatment team, so don't be afraid to ask questions, speak up about side effects, or try another option. Give feedback on your experiences to others, including your caregivers and health providers.

Remember the importance of self-care, and practice it daily. You are the expert on you: no one knows your body or quality of life better than you do. Pain is a good teacher; if you are getting signals that an activity is too painful or you need a break, listen to the message. It is okay to say 'no' to others, to take time for yourself, to avoid activities that exacerbate or induce a flare, and to navigate your own health journey in a manner that is best suited for you and your lifestyle.

Invite your community leaders, legislators, hospitals and local healthcare professionals to become part of your network to learn about the best ways they can help us achieve strides in the disease. Many epidemiological studies have linked measures of social support to physical health outcomes, so be sure to also seek out a quality support system that can guide your journey; one which shares critical resources, accurate facts and disease information, and offers a forum in which to become empowered over endometriosis.

Be an ambassador and lend your own guidance and expertise: if you see someone missing school or work from painful periods or pelvic pain or infertility, talk to them. Correct misinformation when you see it, using quality citations and unbiased, trusted, peer-reviewed information reflecting modern concepts about endometriosis.

Above all else: you do not have to suffer in silence.

Laparoscopic Excision surgery combined with true multidisciplinary approaches to the disease changed my life. Ultimately, adenomyosis did lead to that hysterectomy & bilateral salpingo-oophorectomy twenty years ago, and I will never be "completely well" given my extensive and damaging history with this disease. But I have a miracle child. I am endometriosis-free. I have my life back. I am still here. I no longer keep endometriosis a secret - and you don't have to, either.

My story is far from unique or the worst. I share it only because I want society to know that early access to educated providers and proper treatment can reduce needless suffering. Had I been offered the high-quality, multidisciplinary care I later received earlier on in my odyssey, life may have been very different for me – and can be for countless others now.

Nevertheless, I've been afforded a lifetime filled not only with pain, but more importantly, with countless blessings and the most amazing mentors, teachers, friends and connections as a result of endometriosis. I am proof that our stories don't have to end hopelessly.

We need to help those with endometriosis get well. If we work together to better educate society about early intervention and gold-standard, organ-sparing excisional/multidisciplinary treatment, change our culture of misinformation and societal bias, and throw a lifeline to those struggling, we can make a positive difference. Those impacted by endometriosis deserve as much – and more.

I cannot get back what the disease stole from me, but it's never too late to tell my tale and encourage others down a different path. I share my (many) scars in the hope that it helps someone else from acquiring their own - and because, sometimes, the journey is easier if we go with someone who can light the way. The time for the 'innovation drought' in endometriosis to end has long passed.

Heather Guidone
Program Director
Center for Endometriosis Care, May 2018.

For Nancy, for lighting my journey; for Lou & Dylan, for lighting my world. Dedicated to Ken Sinervo, MD & Robert B. Albee, Jr., MD for saving lives every day, including mine.

> "It threatens EVERY aspect of life, as you may have known it or thought it would have been ..."
>
> – Amy Jane Melhuish

ONE

Amy Jane Melhuish, France

A note from Amy Jane …

It's the pain of endometriosis that's been making me grumpy, not just French bureaucracy.

Hot water-bottles shoved front-and-back down my pyjamas hinders movement to and from anywhere to anywhere. Pain that makes me want to throw up or pass out does its best to steal my focus. Pain, dizziness, bloating, horrific night-sweats and bowel and bladder issues because it's my "period".

This seems very strange to say, seeing as I had a hysterectomy years ago (just one of multiple surgeries since 2005).

I'm a veteran at all of this now at forty years old. The pain started when I was fourteen. It took thirteen years for a diagnosis which was first in 2005. I learned how to still 'do' life. I fight hard, then teach myself. I am lucky enough to have met a gem of a man who is willing to share that life with me - endometriosis and all - that's been a six year journey of acceptance for both of us.

Learning to be loved.

Speaking of love, my cycle meant no lovin' before he went away on a work trip for a week (see aforementioned symptoms, not particularly sexy). I'm ill twice a month, ovulation too. So just a squeeze and some tears shed. I may be a veteran, but it's still hard for him to see me like this, it never gets easier for anyone.

Thankfully, when I messed up my dosage years ago (I've always got ml and cl confused), I had my stomach pumped and am still here to tell the tale. But there are many successful suicides amongst endometriosis sufferers and I understand why. It is a life-threatening disease. It threatens every aspect of life as you may have known it or thought it would have been.

I've been awake since 7 am but unable to move. Thanks to my husband pimping my phone, my day can start from my bed nest.

My diary gets arranged according to my cycle. Last night I had three hours in a hot bath - I don't bother going to A&E anymore as the homecare coping mechanisms I've established are far kinder on my mental, spiritual & emotional wellbeing than the standard accusatory and dismissive reception of overwhelmed hospital staff. Not blaming them (some not all), but I am highlighting very common occurrences and the need for improvements.

There are more than 176 million of us ladies who suffer globally. If you put us all together, we would form the 8th largest country in the world apparently. But I believe that 1 in 10 statistic isn't true either.

To be a statistic you have to have the diagnosis, which still takes an average of eight to ten years, or by being actively treated by a Dr. I stopped all synthetic hormones and meds years ago, because the drugs didn't work and they made me feel worse.

Symptoms are often masked until a lady stops taking The Pill ...and then has pain and/or infertility issues come into focus. Endometriosis outside the gynae region is not rare. Finding medical professionals who understand that however, is rare. That is not the same thing.

Time's up on women's health 'care'. Things have to change.

"Oooo you look tanned!" my doctor says…

No, I'm flushed in pain, done with falling apart, everything is actually finally falling into place.

About Amy Jane

From their old stone house in the South of France, Amy Jane helps women of all ages to be chronically awesome and lead the life they desire, their own.

Picture Mary Poppins meets Rosie the Riveter. A duffle bag full of questionable humour, warm smiles, tough love, free-form food, the odd power tool, a bit of woo, strategic thinking, heat pads...and probably gin.

Amy Jane has led a full and interesting life. One that has had many plot twists along the way. In realising things haven't changed for the most part across the decades she's suffered - and quite frankly sick of the pain and corruption - she is drawing on her business experience and grit and making it her mission to launch EndoGate™ as soon as humanly possible promising to be a global portal and information highway between true endo specialists, researchers, and support groups to those on the ground.

EndoGate™ Because time's up on taboo and time's most certainly up on the farce of women's healthcare. Poisonous protocols don't work. Outdated information isn't helping. Women deserve better.

For more information about EndoGate™□, Amy Jane, endometriosis and more: If you're keen for you or your organisation to be included in EndoGate™, would like to pledge your support for the project, or to be kept up-to-date with the latest, then email amy.melhuish@gmail.com or messenger Amy Jane Melhuish via Facebook.

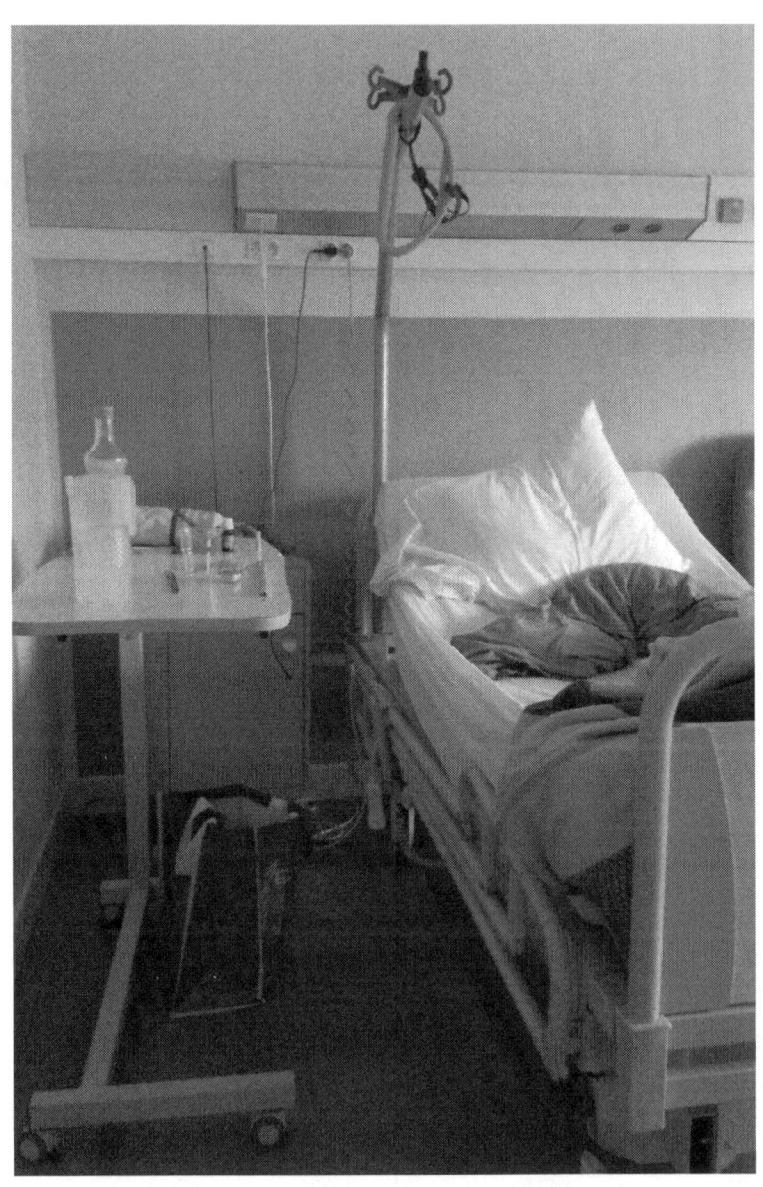

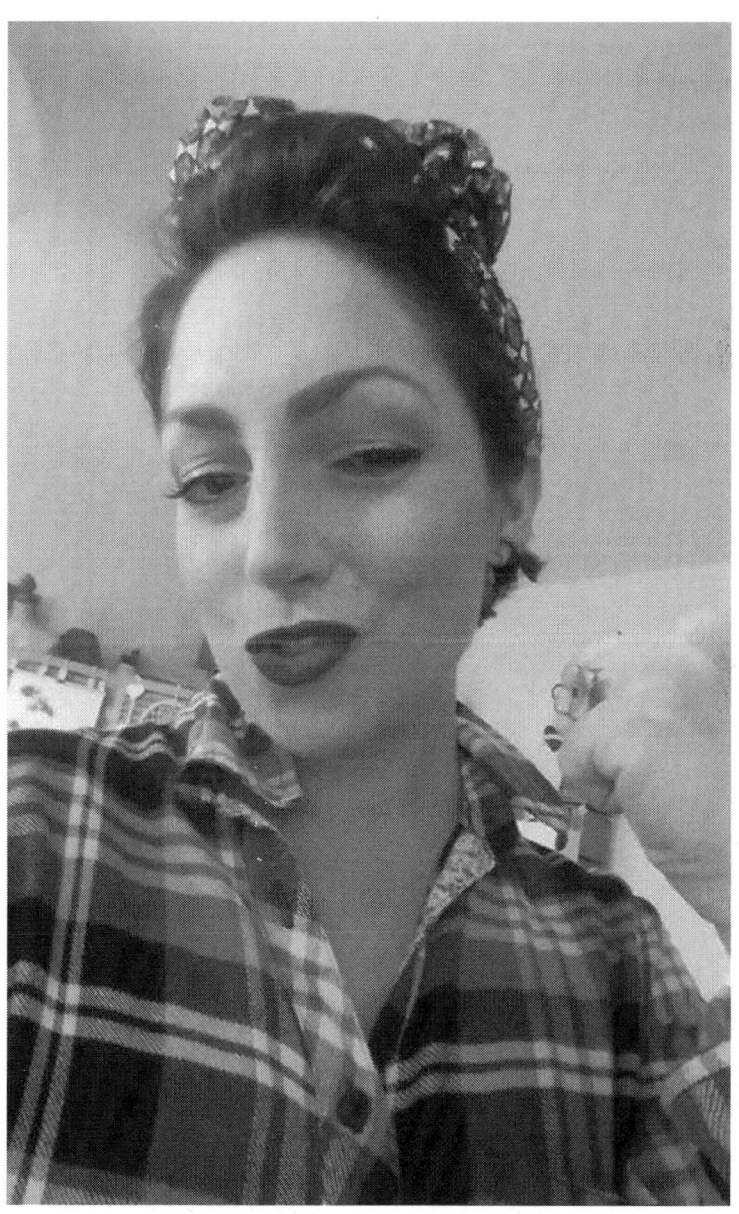

"I'm not even sure how to approach this, but I have endometriosis and I've had it for 22 years."

– Allenia Owens

TWO

Allenia Owens, California

I'm not even sure how to approach this but I have endometriosis and I've had it for twenty-two years.

Most days I wake up exhausted, because there's something spreading inside my body that sucks all of my energy all day long.

The pain, when it comes is phenomenal and so deep that I have found ways to detach my mind from my body. There are days I can't eat, sleep, move, or just be a normal person and enjoy things like work or socializing. It's a terrorizing and debilitating disease.

I went so far as to have a hysterectomy on March 18, 2016 knowing damn well it wouldn't cure my endometriosis but so desperately needing to stop the pain. For that, I sacrificed my little chance to have children.

I hate endometriosis.

The pain and destruction of my organs continues, but I will not let it ruin me. It's barely starting to be recognized for the awful condition/disease that it is. I'm "1 in 10" women fighting for some help and I just want you to know there 176 million of us fighting for the same thing: a pain-free, productive, enjoyable, normal life that doesn't revolve around this damn disease.

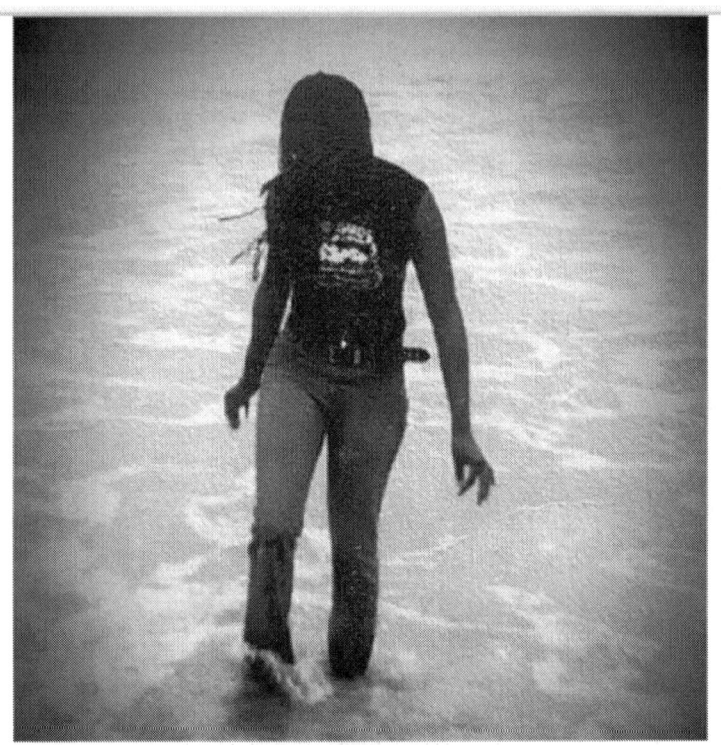

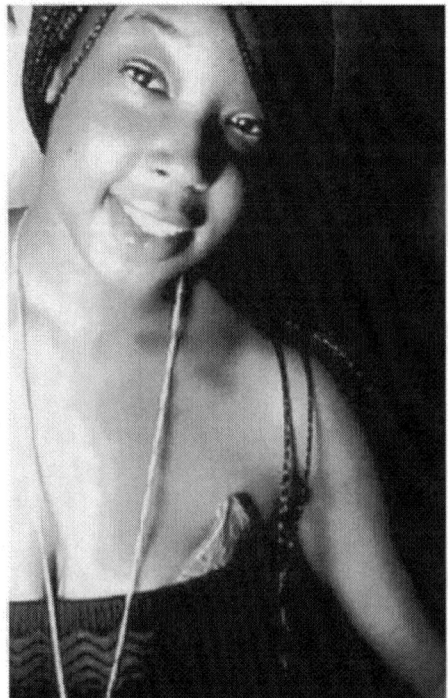

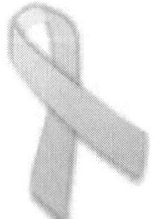

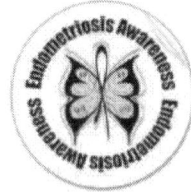

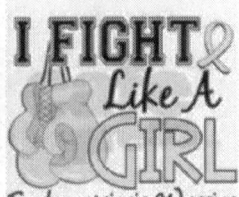

"This disease causes head-to-toe issues. Very few have only endometriosis."

– Stephanie Parido

THREE

Stephanie Parido, California

March is Endometriosis Awareness Month

My symptoms started in my late 20's I was first diagnosed with the sister-disease, interstitial cystitis, at 29 years old. I ignored my symptoms as they were five to seven days a month until I suffered a chocolate cyst at 41. This led to a added diagnosis of adenomyosis and stage 4 endometriosis.

My doctor was not qualified and he aspirated my cyst when it needed to be cut out, I was back in surgery one year later and of course much worse.

I started looking for a top doctor. I traveled for partial hysterectomy (which only cures adenomyosis), excision (endometriosis cutting at root), and appendectomy (endometriosis was all over my appendix). My ovary by this time was overtaken by the cyst, so the left one was removed but it was also suck to my bowel.

I went into surgical menopause at 44 years old. Four years later I now have seventeen different chronic illnesses and still diagnosing more. This disease causes head to toe issues, very few have only endometriosis. Endo is very common however, every story is unique, every woman deals with it differently.

My message is simple. Do not ignore symptoms. Maybe my story would have turned out differently if I had gotten a diagnose when I first started having symptoms. Maybe.

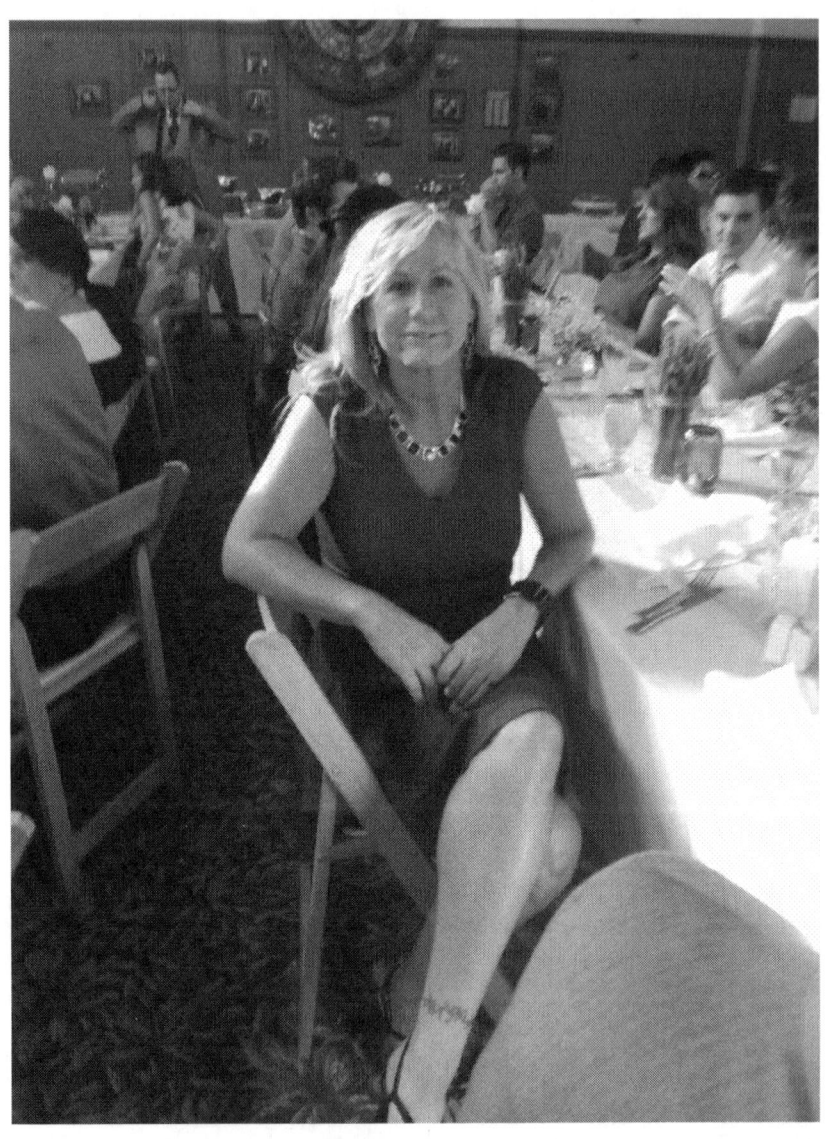

> "I almost died at 26 years old, because I was conditioned to believe pelvic pain was a normal part of being female."
>
> – Renee Papesh

FOUR

Renee Papesh (RN), Wisconsin

August 2009 was a wonderful and terrifying time for me and my family.

Our son was born on the 5th, our first wedding anniversary was the 16th, and then I was admitted to the ICU on the 18th. Postpartum uterine infection... sepsis.

I almost died at 26 years old because I was conditioned to believe pelvic pain was a normal part of being female. I had undiagnosed and very symptomatic endometriosis & adenomyosis. My uterus was dysfunctional and this was ignored despite my questions.

My husband almost lost me, he was almost left to care for two small babies by himself because of medical misogyny.

Postpartum Pain:

I had a terrible time being pregnant and giving birth to both of my children. As it turns out, I had undiagnosed endometriosis. Endometriosis is different for everyone and not all will have infertility, but many develop complications during pregnancy and delivery. I had a lot of digestive dysfunction, crushing fatigue, pelvic pain and kidney pain during my pregnancies, not to mention my obliterated pelvic floor.

After the birth of my son, I really did not feel well. I was exhausted and crampy, my back was so pained and my head pounded. My doctor assured me that I was just tired and sore from having a baby, and that maybe I should get some rest. Did I mention we lived on an island? The hospital was an hour away, including the thirty minute ferry boat ride. I rested. I pushed fluids. I got worse.

Three weeks postpartum and two days after my first wedding anniversary, I insisted on going to the ER. I was nauseated, dizzy, and weak. I couldn't stand without extreme pain, I could no longer lift my infant, and my breasts had become two flaming hot rocks despite my nursing and pumping efforts. I felt like I was dying.

We made it to the hospital only to be chastised by the doctor. Why hadn't we called our primary first? Didn't we know mastitis wasn't a medical emergency? There I was, a 26-year-old female medicaid patient, about to be discharged when my nurse insisted there was something else going on. My blood pressure was dropping, even after the bolus of fluids, my heart rate soared into the 120 range, and the room was going dim. A flurry of people whirled around the bed.

A blood culture and tortuous pelvic exam revealed postpartum endometritis and septicemia, the sort of thing women in the 1800s died from regularly. I spent three days in the ICU with a three week old newborn and not-yet-two year old at home. My children almost lost their mother and I almost lost my life.

It took three more years of pain beyond description to persuade a doctor to perform exploratory surgery. I was diagnosed with stage IV endometriosis. It was everywhere: colon, rectum, cul-de-sac, vagina, ovaries, bladder, ureter, peritoneum, ligaments, sacrum, and adenomyosis (endo of the uterus). I have had four surgeries in five years, I have only one remaining ovary, and I remain in chronic pain. It does not have to be this way.

Pelvic pain is never normal.

We can no longer culture girls and women to accept that pain is normal part of womanhood, of femaleness. This is a dangerous lie. When female pain is discredited and dismissed the consequences can be deadly.

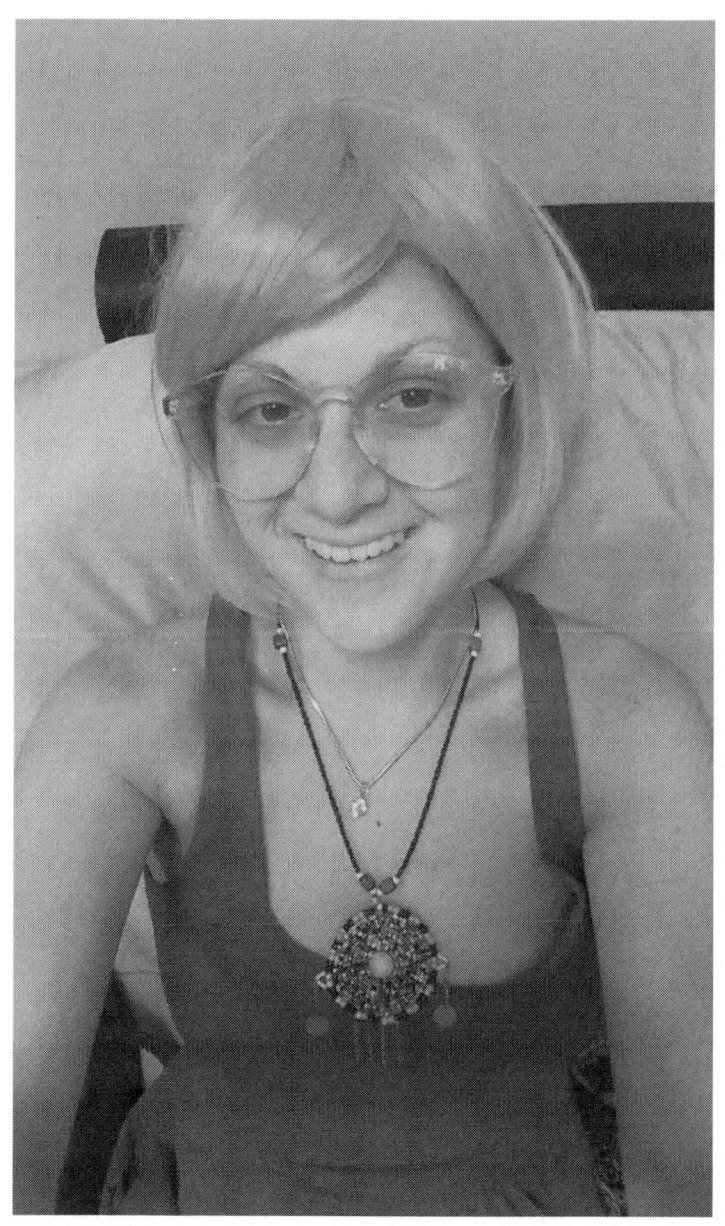

"It was all wrapped around my bowels and it cost me my fertility."

– Joy Grey

FIVE

Joy Grey, South Carolina

My goal is to educate others about Endometriosis. You are not alone. I ask that you don't give up no matter how exhausted you are.

Here is my story ...

In 2003 I married the most amazing man. Little did I know how amazing he was really going to be. "For Better or For Worse." Yeah that's what we meant.

I was diagnosed with endometriosis in 2004. It was all wrapped around my bowels and it caused me not to be able to have children, but on a good note I was blessed with the adoption of our son Blake.

My Endo came back a few years ago and moved in my upper body. Who knew that could happen? Not me. My Obgyn insisted this couldn't happen. Yeah, right!

I'm learning more and more about this disease everyday. I have had five surgeries for endometriosis. My first in 2004, my second in November 2015. My Obgyn attempted a hysterectomy. He said it was the worst surgery he had ever performed. My whole pelvis was frozen. He had to chisel to get to what he could. Knowing my history he should have referred me to a specialist a lot sooner.

After my hysterectomy I continued to get worse. Finally I received my referral and was scheduled to have my third surgery on May 12th 2016, but this time with Dr. Sinervo. Surgery took over seven hours.

I knew instantly my endometriosis was gone, but unfortunately I didn't know the damage. After returning home on the 20th I was on a plane again returning to Atlanta for my fourth round, this time to add a bag due to a fistula. I spent most of my summer in and out of hospitals. I missed my birthday, my son's and even my dad's. Bowel blockages, picc lines, nose tubes and home health nurses. TPN became my friend that is I was fed intravenously. Everytime I tried to eat or drink I ended up with a bowel blockage.

I had what I am hoping was my final surgery in August to correct the bowel blockage. Unfortunately I came home and ended up with another fistula. Back to adult diapers again.

I was scheduled to have my sixth surgery this past December, but this time the fistula healed on its own. Valentine's Day 2017 I started physical therapy on my diaphragm. Soon I will start pelvic therapy.

One day at a time, one foot in front of the other.

The last couple of weeks I have finally started to feel better, even catching up on my sleep. Walking up to three miles when at one time I could barely make it down my sidewalk.

My recommendation to you...please please please do more research and make sure you are in the hands of a surgeon who can take care of this disease the way it should be taken care of.

A huge thank you first and foremost to my Lord and Savior Jesus Christ. He blessed me with Dr. Ken Sinervo and his team at The Center for Endometriosis Care out of Atlanta, Georgia. How great it was to have a surgeon hold my hand and pray with me before each surgery. I have always been used to being asleep before I got to the operating room. Not with Dr Sinervo.

I sure wish our paths would have crossed in 2004. Yeah right.

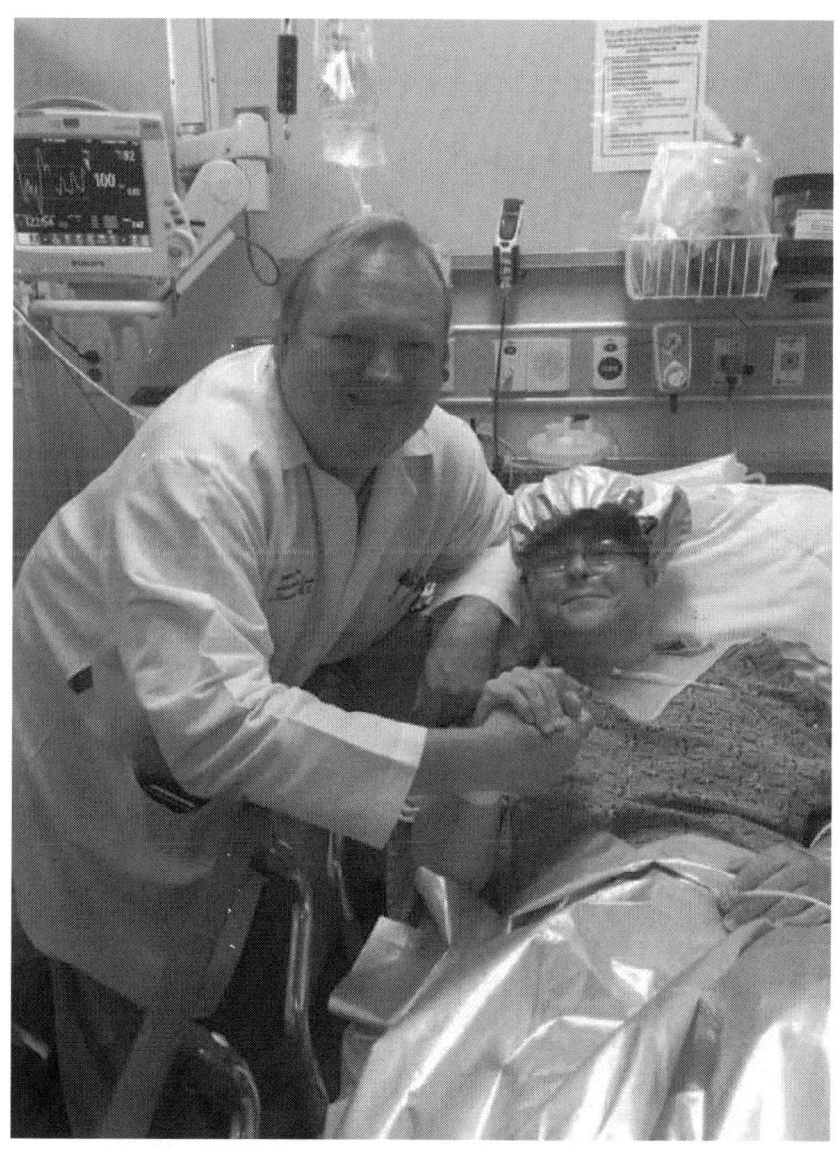

"My doctor told me I was Stage 3, which is moderate. If I was at Stage 4, she said, she would have to do a full hysterectomy on me. I was only 16 years old at the time."

– Alyssa Sanchez

SIX

Alyssa Sanchez, New York

So since it's endometriosis awareness month and I get asked all the time about it, so I decided to share my story.

By thirteen years old, every other week it seemed like I was in the hospital complaining of horrible stomach pain, bleeding so bad, sobbing my eyes out. No matter what they gave me, it wouldn't fix anything. But the thing is, these episodes would only happen during my cycle. Right then and there I knew something wasn't right or normal.

I finally had the courage to go see a gynecologist. I had testing done. A lot of testing. Bloodwork, sonogram and MRI. My bloodwork came back normal. So did the sonogram. The MRI, however, showed a mass-type substance.

My doctor was very concerned, because she couldn't rule out whether it was cancer. So on top of all the other stuff i had to go through, I needed to have tumor markers to rule out cancer. That had to be scariest thing I ever had to go through.

Luckily everything came back normal. It wasn't cancer. My doctor recommended that I have a laparoscopy, which is exploratory surgery. Because of the pain I was in she thought it was best to do that to take a peek inside.

She suggested the pain i was in and other issues I was having showed signs of endometriosis. Nothing more was said or explained to me what it was, just that it could be a suggestion of a possibility of what's causing all my issues.

Bump it to my first surgery. My lap surgery and diagnosis surgery. I woke up to my doctor hugging me tight saying you're one lucky girl. "Why?" I asked. She said. "Alyssa this is hard for me to tell you this, but your insides were completely covered in endometriosis and that mass we saw on the test was your ovary enlarged."

She proceeded to tell me she had to cut open my right ovary and out came a chocolate cyst. Then started to explain to me exactly what endometriosis really was.

There is no cure for endo, it does not show up in any tests and the only way to see it is to be opened up. My doctor said that I have a huge battle ahead of me. She also told me I was at stage 3 which is moderate. If I had been at stage 4, she would have had to do a full hysterectomy on me. I was only sixteen at the time. The looks on my family's faces and the sound of cries in my room is something that will be buried in my head forever.

Since then, I've had a total of eight endometriosis surgeries in almost four years. Most of them about seven months apart from another. I've had my gallbladder and appendix removed because of my endometriosis. My endo was actually so bad at one point that it pushed my appendix all the way up to where it was sitting under my breast. It took the surgeon fifteen minutes just to find it.

I decided to do the Lupron and depo shots to help keep the endo under control. Like I said previously, there's no cure just harsh medicine to help get it under control. Lupron is chemo that they actually use to help with prostate cancer and we all know what the depo consists of.

I gained so much weight. Fell into deep depression. Many times i wanted to just end my life, because I couldn't take being on the medicine, the pain of endo and the countless surgeries.

I also developed severe anxiety. Everything just seemed to be falling apart. I developed osteoporosis because of my medication, had hair loss and also vitamin deficiency. I went through hell being on the depo. It caused me to have severe pressure in my head all day every day and I needed a spinal tap done and infusions. I'm currently off the depo for good.

Endo has robbed me from everything. It's like I'm creating a whole new life and I had to cope with it. Everyone is always asking me what does endo feel like. It's hard to explain, but I often say: Have a bad cramp? Multiply that by ten, and then imagine having to live that way all day, every day. It's like someone wrapped barbed wire around my belly and keeps tugging it tightening around my belly. The pain is indescribable.

It's been a long journey and still is. Without the love and support I have, I wouldn't be able to make it through all that I have to go through. If you don't like what you read or feel like it's TMI, feel free to move along. I'm not doing this for pity. I'm doing this to show people this is the reality of living life with endo.

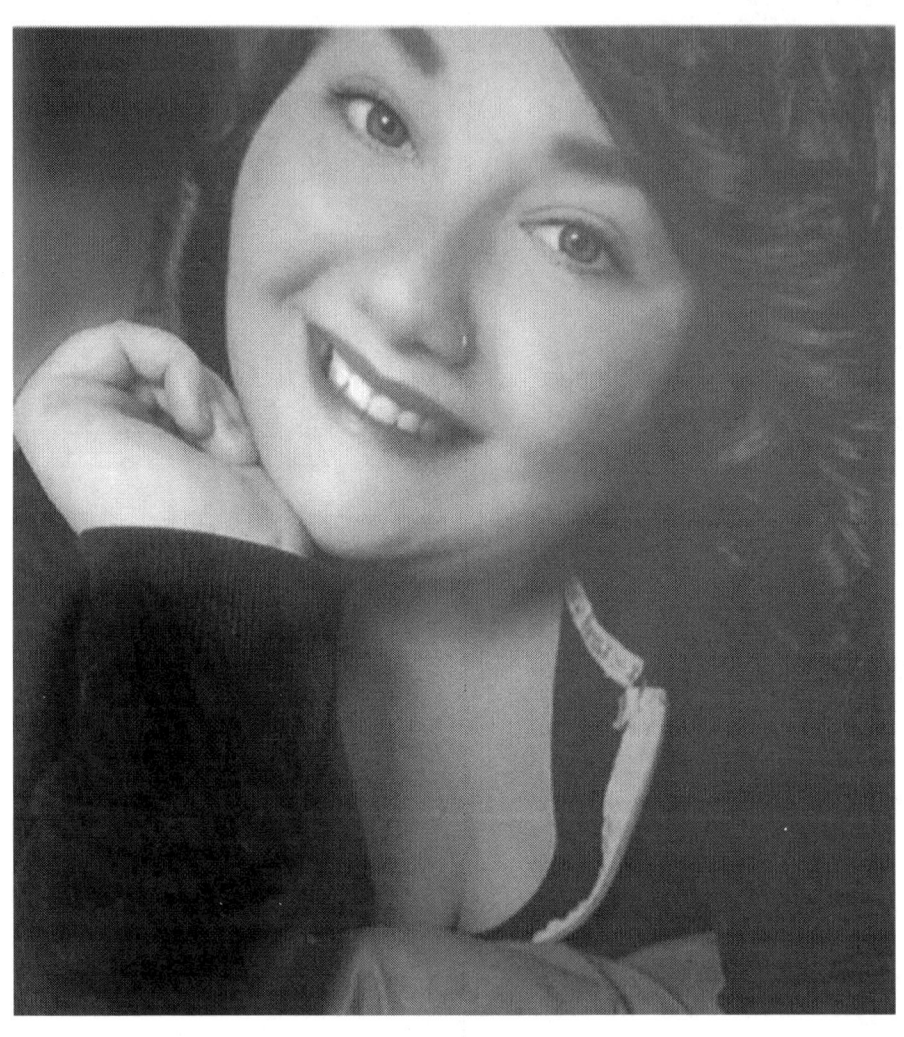

> "A part of me feels bad for forgetting how painful it can be. How could I ever forget?"
>
> – Anna Gaboury

SEVEN

Anna Gaboury, Canada

A personal battle. A painful reminder.

Friday, 2 March 2018:

I missed my birth control pill last Tuesday night. I've been on continuous birth control since my surgery last year and have only taken a few breaks for periods.

Well, I've been spotting on and off since missing my pill and have been having suffering brutal cramps. So bad that I'm confident my endometriosis is back.

It's been a long while since I've felt this excruciating pain inside. It's like knives stabbing, with hot pokers and someone pulling on your insides all at once. I hate this disease so much.

I know I should probably break for a period too, but it's just not something I want to deal with in my life right now, and doubt I could handle it well at all right now. I can't afford to be an emotional mess. It's just not in the cards, this pain is bad enough.

A part of me feels bad about it too, for forgetting how painful it can be. How could I ever forget?

Even just putting a small tampon in hurts like hell. I had to because the spotting/bleeding is that bad. It's just a nightmare. I'm doing my best to do my aromatherapy to help and taking ibuprofen accordingly. I just hope it ends soon, especially by Wednesday when I have to work.

This pain has a way of putting me in a terrible mood, so bad that I struggle to like myself sometimes. This disease makes me angry – the lack of awareness, the lack of 'treatment', the lack of specialists and just the fact that it affects 1 in 10 women, and yet the healthcare system is so lax in properly treating these women.

We are pinned as fakers, or dismissed because there is no way to see the cause of the pain without proper surgery. It doesn't show up on a CT scan or ultrasound. We are pinned as drug seekers because of this.

I am one in ten women with this condition.

About Me

I'm Anna. I love to make art. Painting is my favourite, I feel like I could paint forever. I also like drawing/sketching, watercolour pencil crayons, permanent markers (I prefer Bic over Sharpies, they have a better tip and last longer). I like to play with different mediums like using Crayola markers and using water with them, collaging, using ink and a nib pen. I also enjoy making jewelry, sewing and cooking and baking.

Anna Gaboury,

Endo blog writer, http://annasendo.blogspot.com

Admin, Endometriosis support for Durham region.

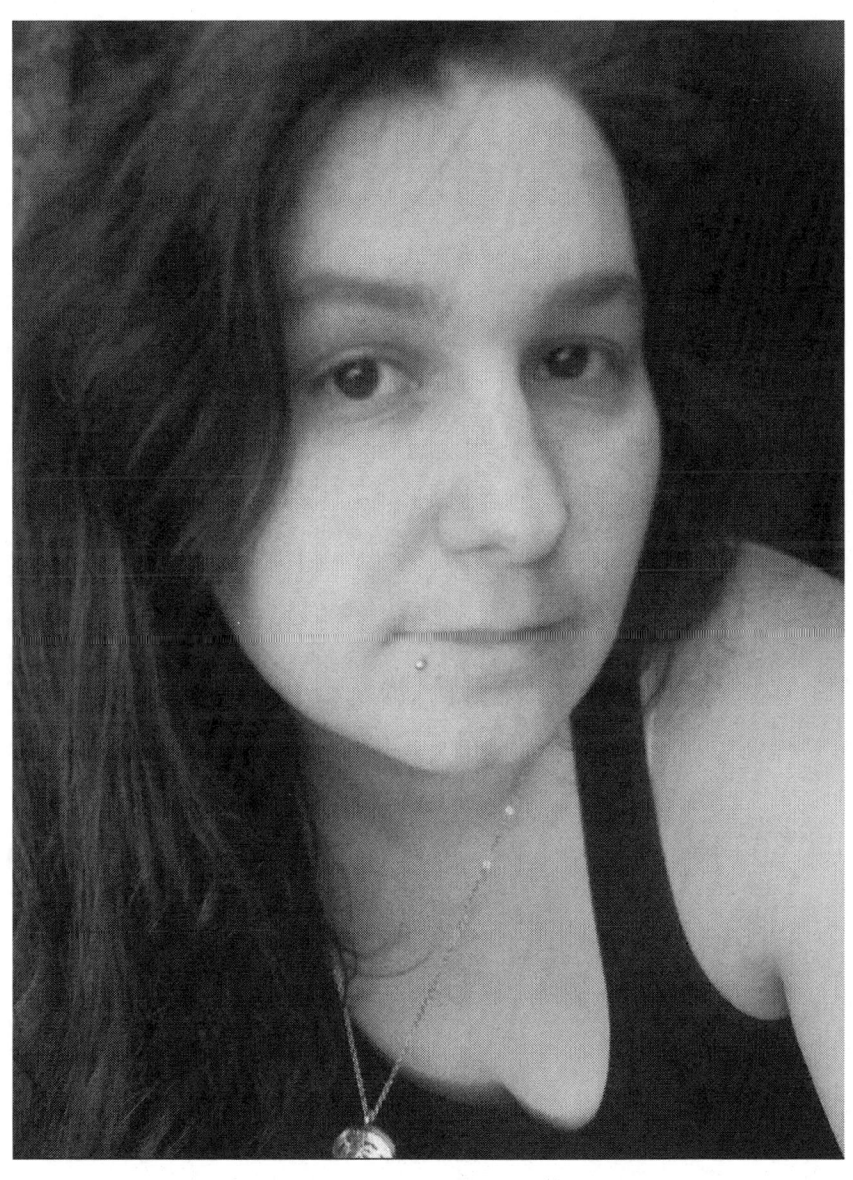

"Despite having four separate surgeons investigate my pelvis laparoscopically, I was not aware I had a severe disease impacting multiple organs until I saw an endo specialist."

– Casey Berna

EIGHT

Casey Berna, MSW, North Carolina

The Cost and Price of Endometriosis

It took me 13 years to get diagnosed with endometriosis.

I had four pelvic surgeries before I finally had surgery with an expert endometriosis excision surgeon.

Despite having four separate surgeons investigate my pelvis laparoscopically, I was not aware I had severe disease impacting multiple organs until I saw a specialist.

I ultimately needed two excision surgeries and participate in ongoing multidisciplinary care.

I am grateful to be able to have the quality of life that I have today, a life that I once did not think possible.

The truth is, unaware doctors who meant well failed me and prolonged my suffering.

My story is not unique and it is the story of 176 million worldwide. The current medical system is failing patients, especially in the United States.

The American College of Gynecologists and Obstetrics who create the standards of care for endometriosis have been failing patients for decades.

The American Society of Reproductive Medicine who create the standards of care that help endometriosis patients who are also struggling with infertility are also failing patients.

There are countless other medical organizations that too miss the opportunity to educate their providers time and time again.

These medical organizations have been told by advocates and experts that they are failing endometriosis patients. These medical organizations are aware of the prolonged suffering that patients endure because of the failures of their members.

Yet, the cycle of delayed diagnosis, misdiagnosis, and mistreatment continues.

If patients could give a comparable amount of money that influential pharmaceutical companies give to medical organizations, hospitals, providers, researchers, medical journals, endometriosis and women's health non-profits, endometriosis thought leaders, and politicians would that finally change our fates and get us quick access to the support and treatments we need?

How much would we need to raise and disperse to these influential, powerful entities, to not lose our kidneys, our bowels, our uteruses, our fertility, our educational and job opportunities, our sexual, social, emotional, and physical health?

We know the high cost of this disease. It's only fair they name their price.

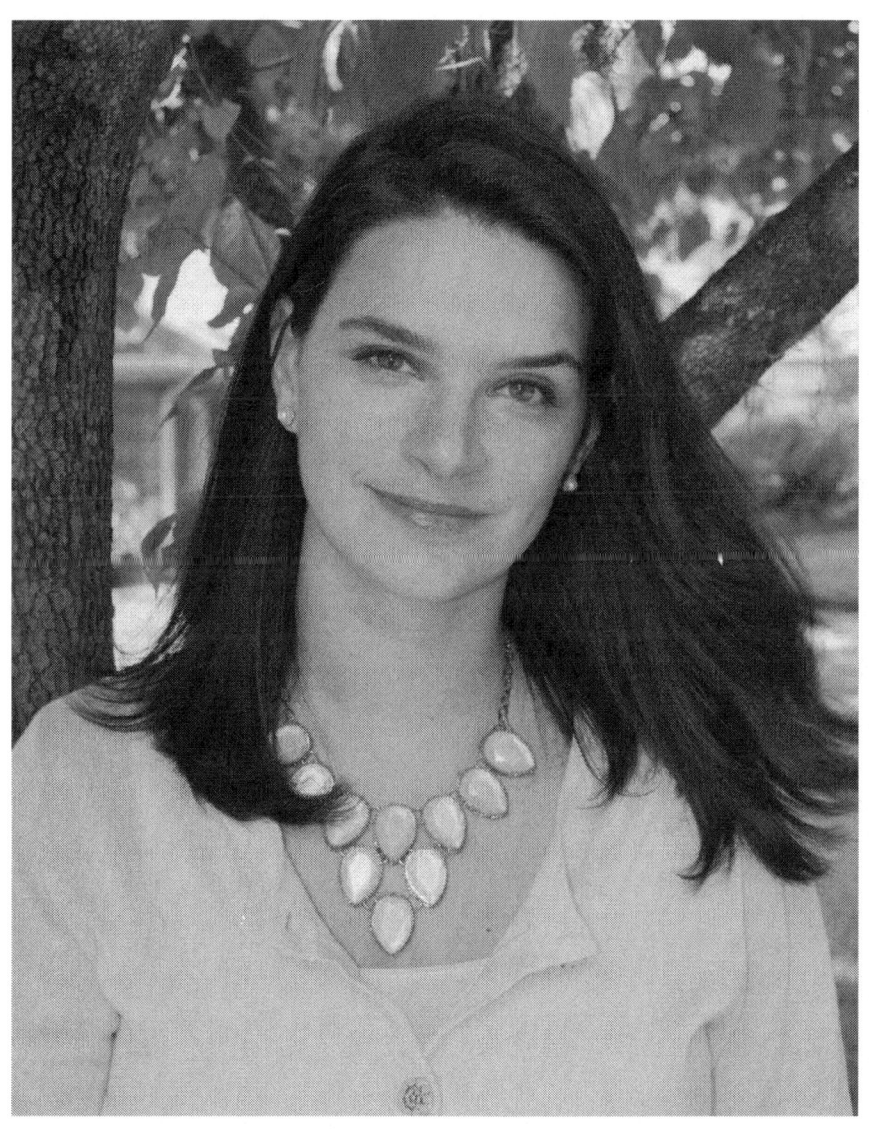

"I hate endometriosis."

— Stephanie Sauer

NINE

Stephanie Saure, California

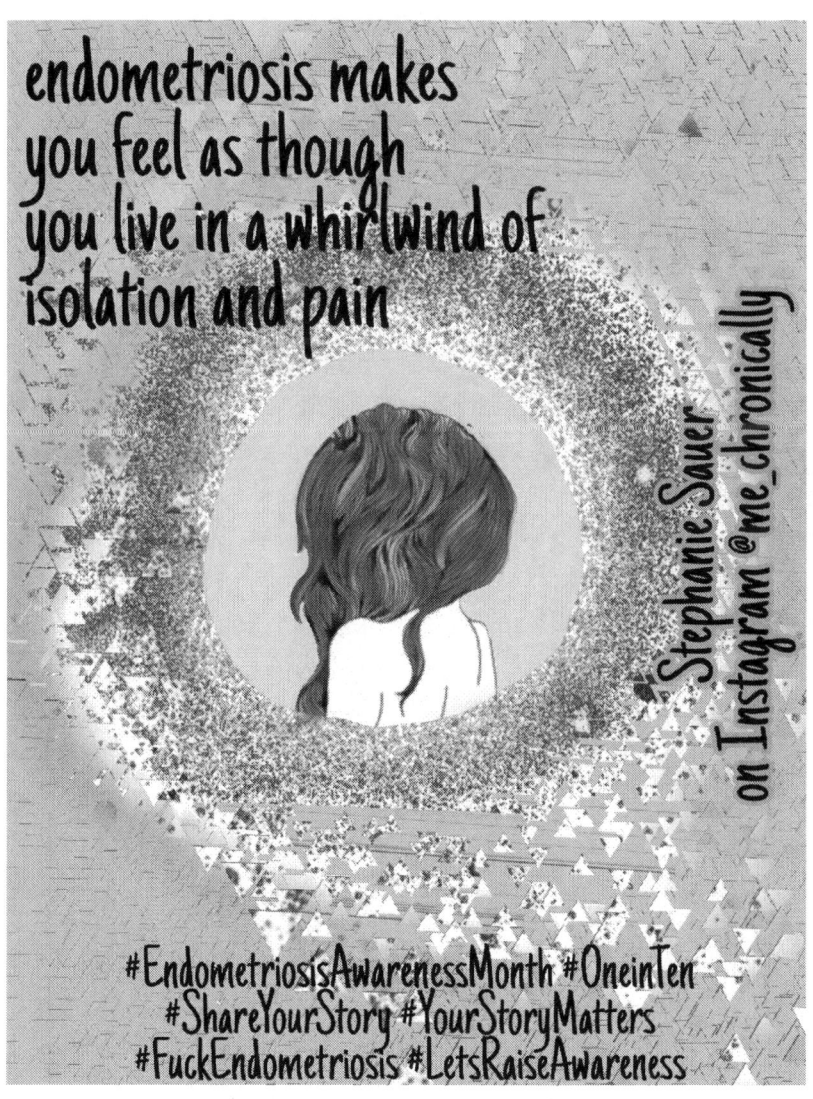

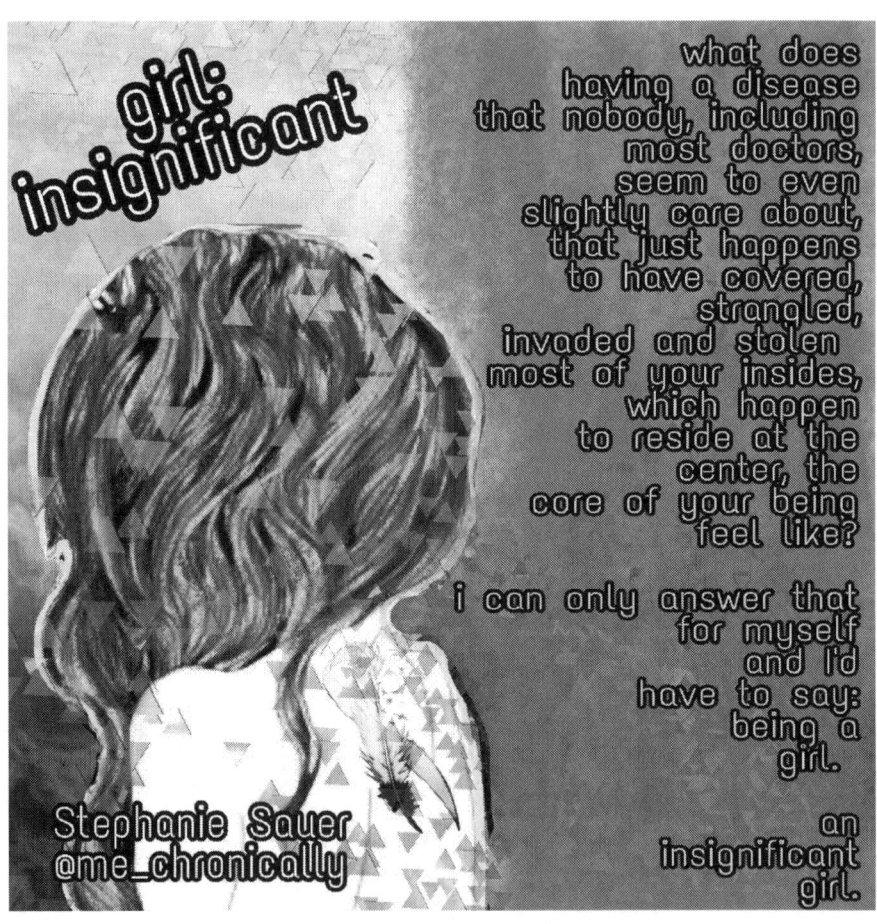

endometriosis awareness

Stephanie Sauer @me_chronically

I used to think I had endometriosis
...
however now I know that
endometriosis has me

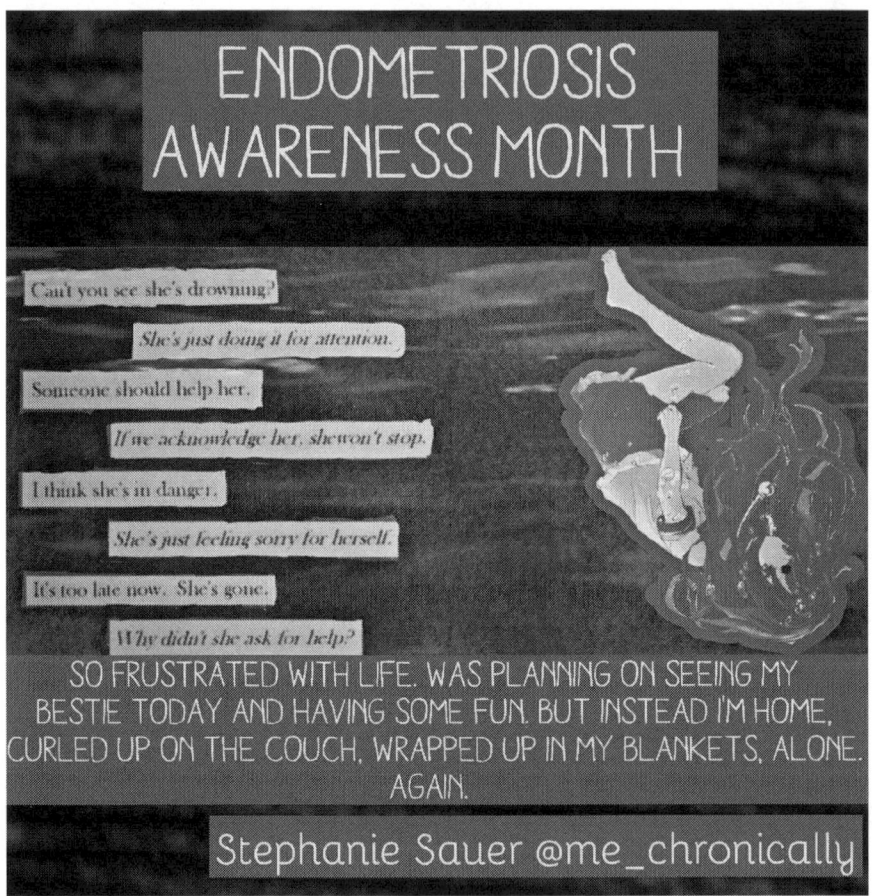

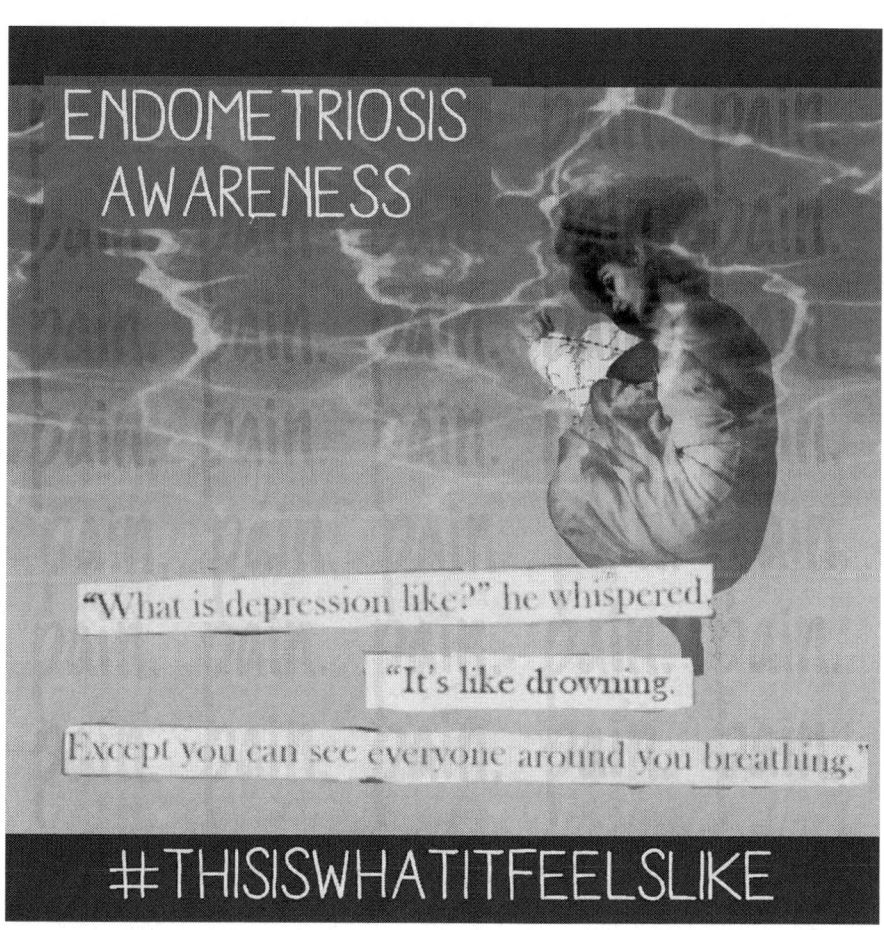

ENDOMETRIOSIS AWARENESS

Most people have standards of how they will be treated in different relationships and how much they are willing to put up with or subject themselves to...
What are you supposed to do if the most abusive relationship you are in is with your very own body?!
In no other aspect of your life would you be willing to be treated in such a horrendous way, resulting in being so viciously abused: physically, emotionally, spiritually, mentally, socially, financially, professionally, psychologically.

Stephanie Sauer

#ENDOMETRIOSISAWARENESS #IAMONEINTEN #SHAREYOURSTORY #YOURSTORYMATTERS #FUCKENDOMETRIOSIS #LETSRAISEAWARENESS

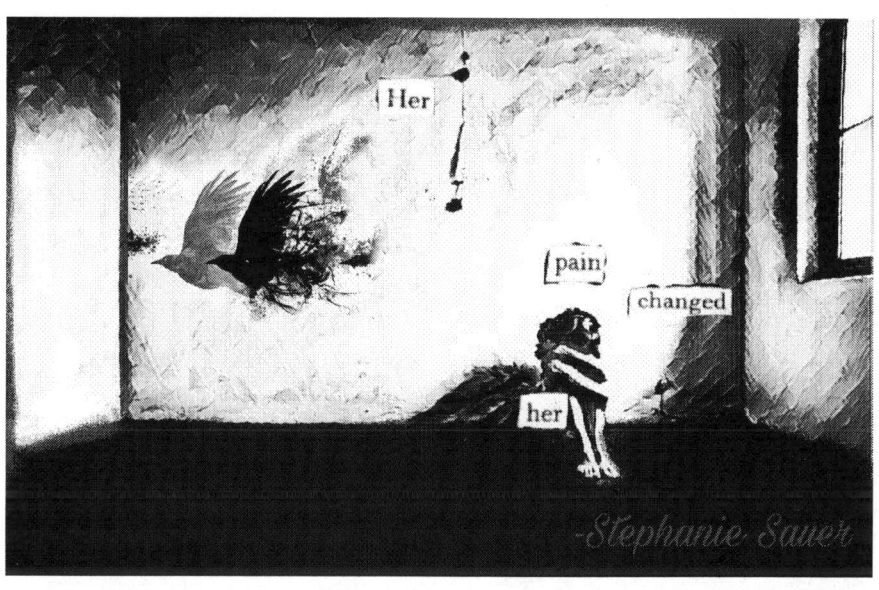

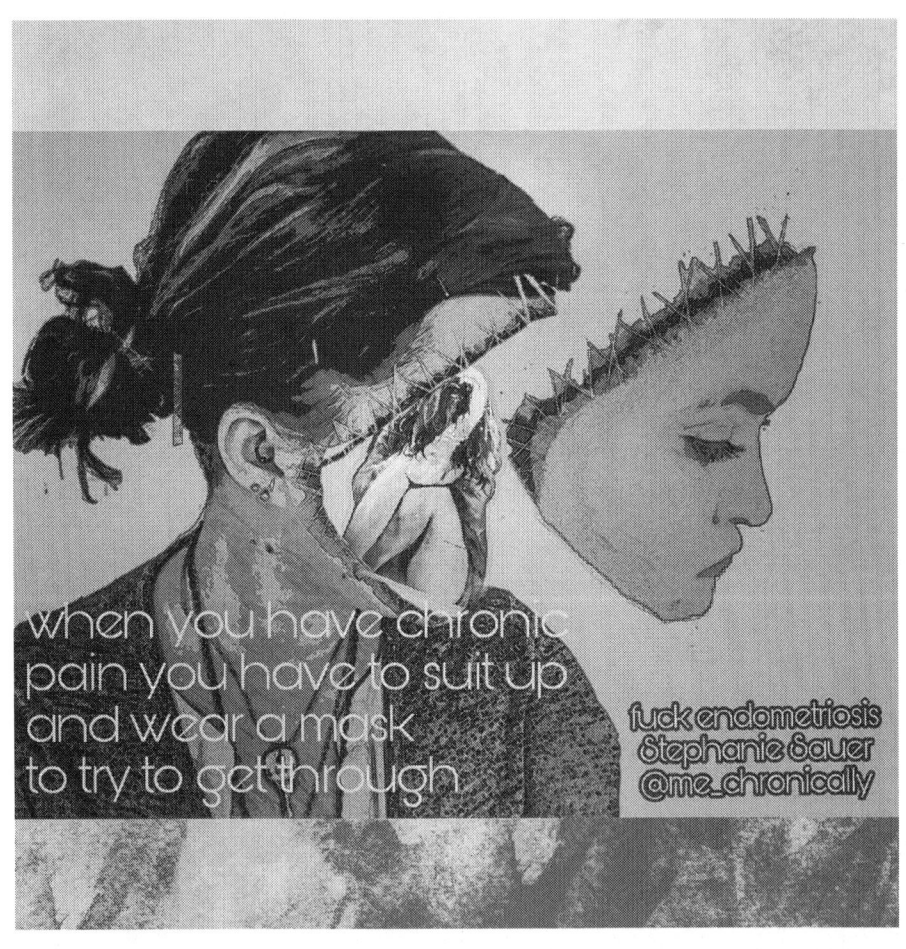

ENDOMETRIOSIS AWARENESS MONTH

endometriosis frequently results in looking quite bloated which can lead to some uncomfortable experiences with people thinking I'm pregnant so while i may look pregnant, just know that this is in fact how i feel. so if you have someone in your life who may appear pregnant, yet you don't know for sure that she is, THINK BEFORE YOU SPEAK, PLEASE.

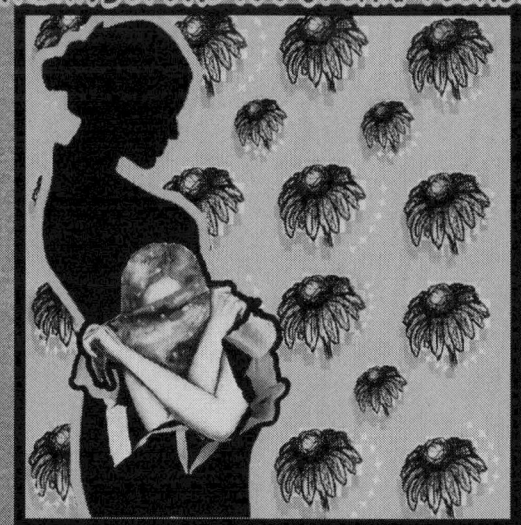

#Endometriosis #Iamlin10 #ShareYourStory #YourStoryMatters #FuckEndometriosis

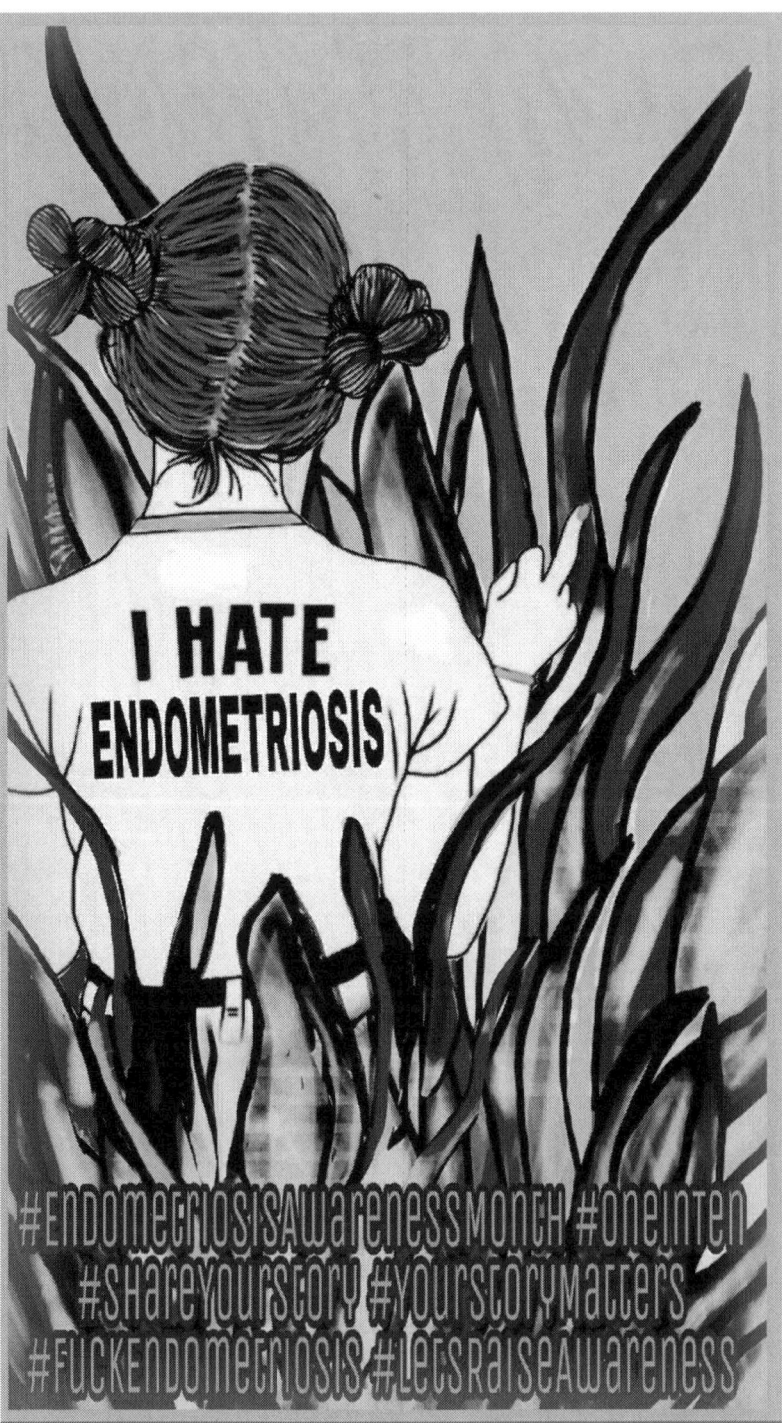

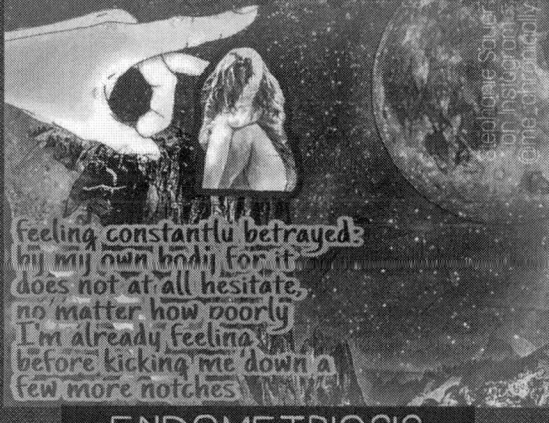

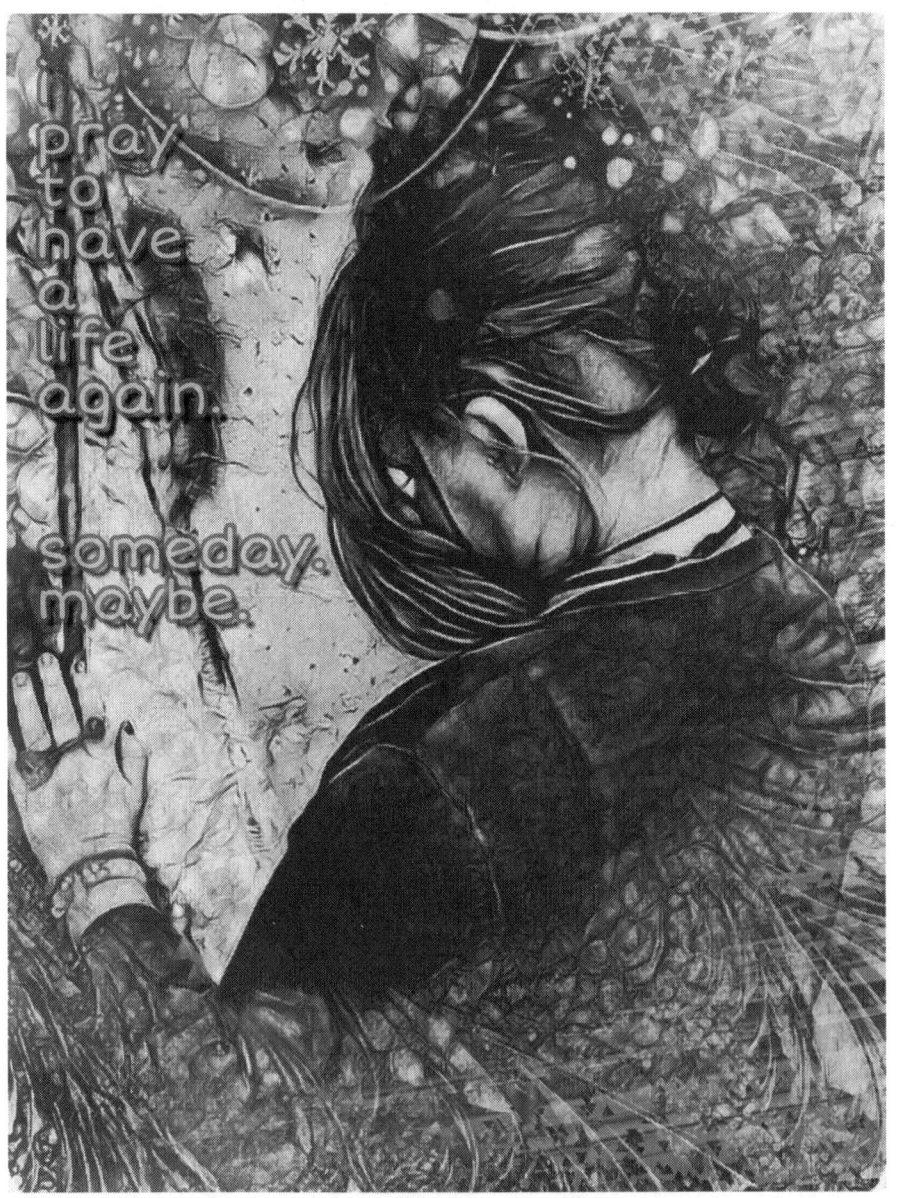

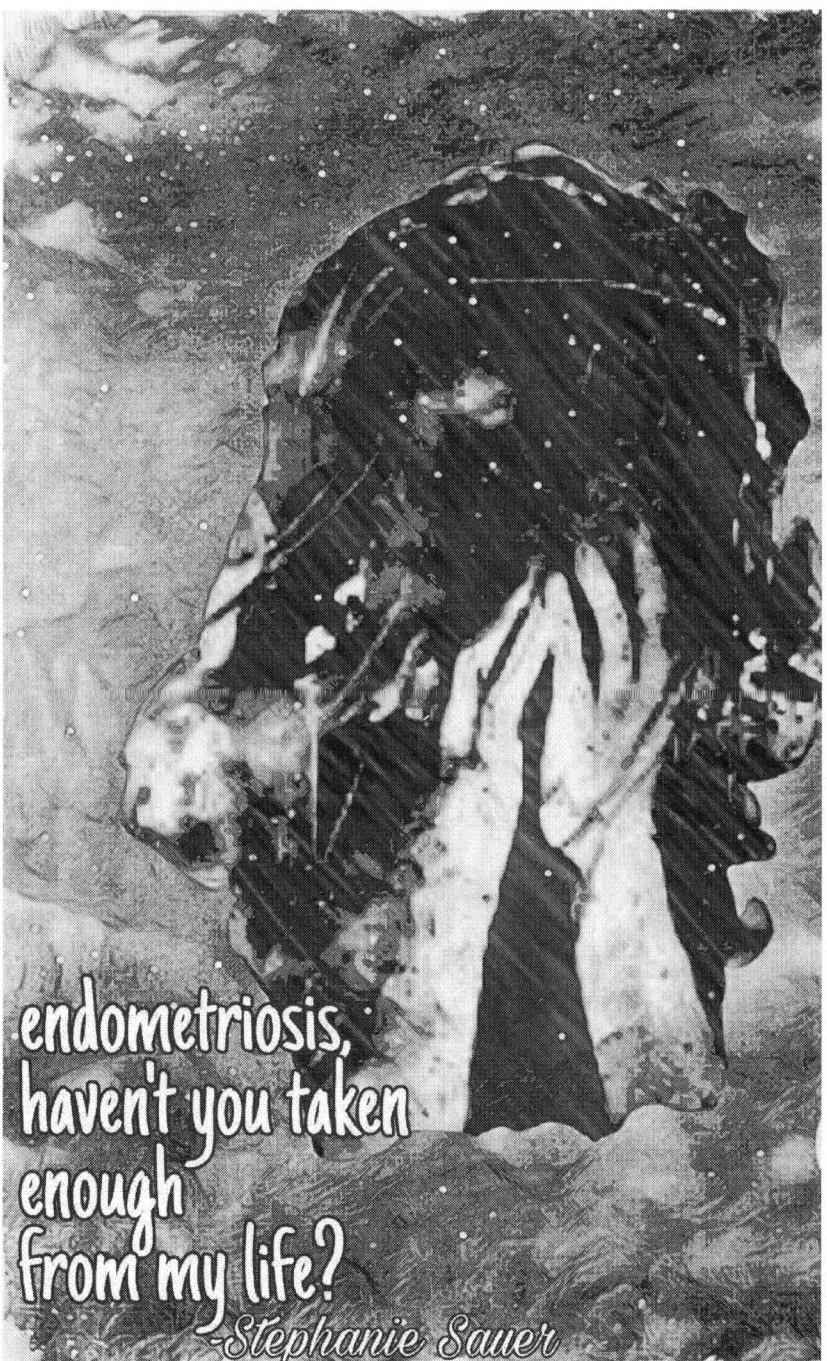

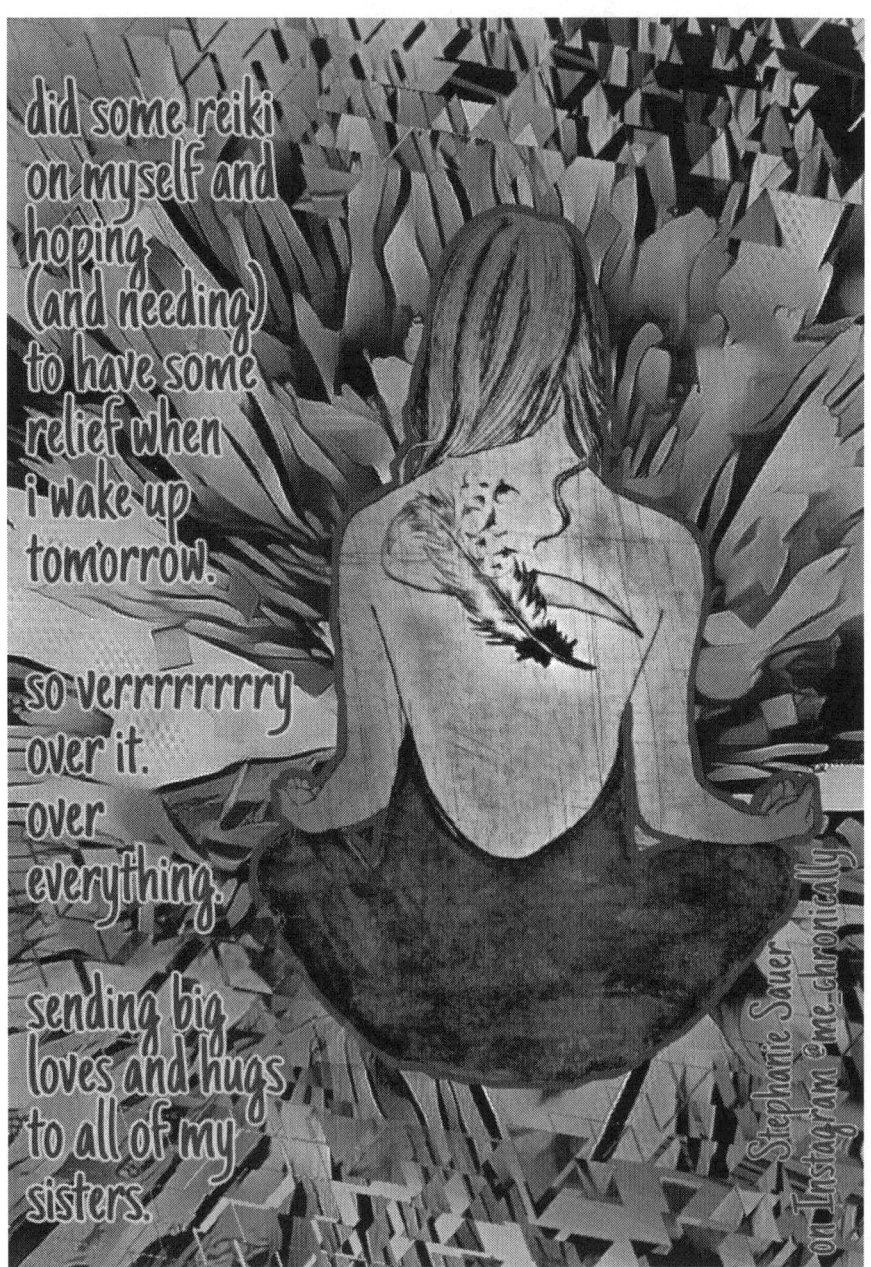

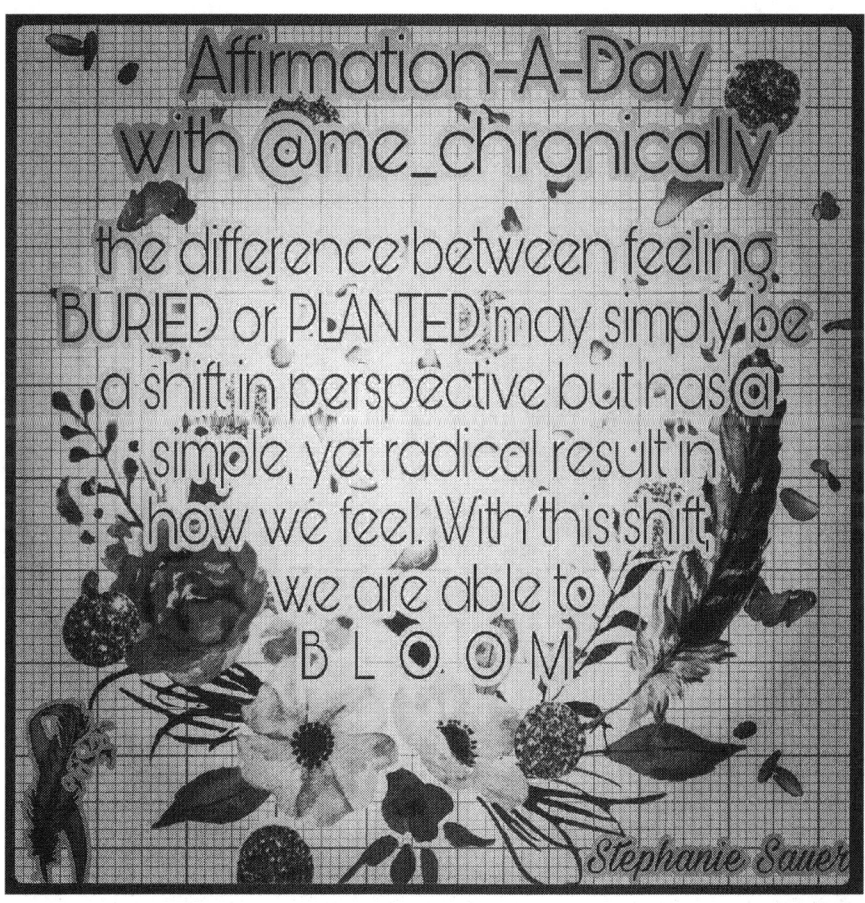

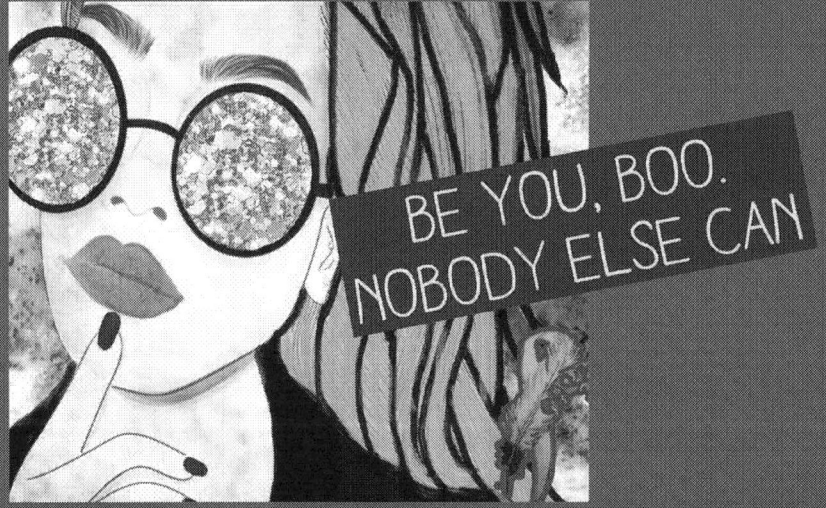

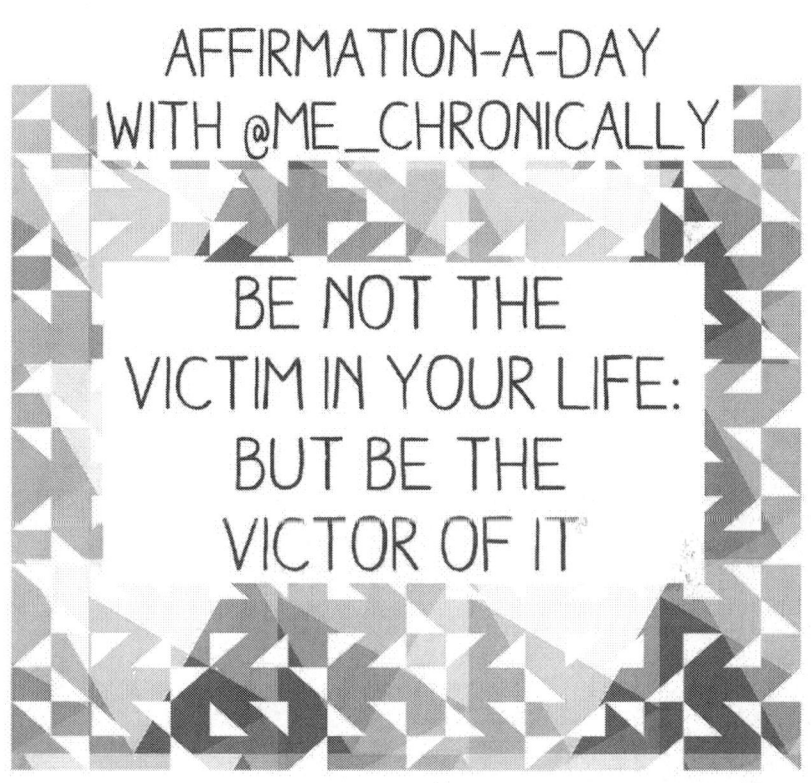

Stephanie Sauer

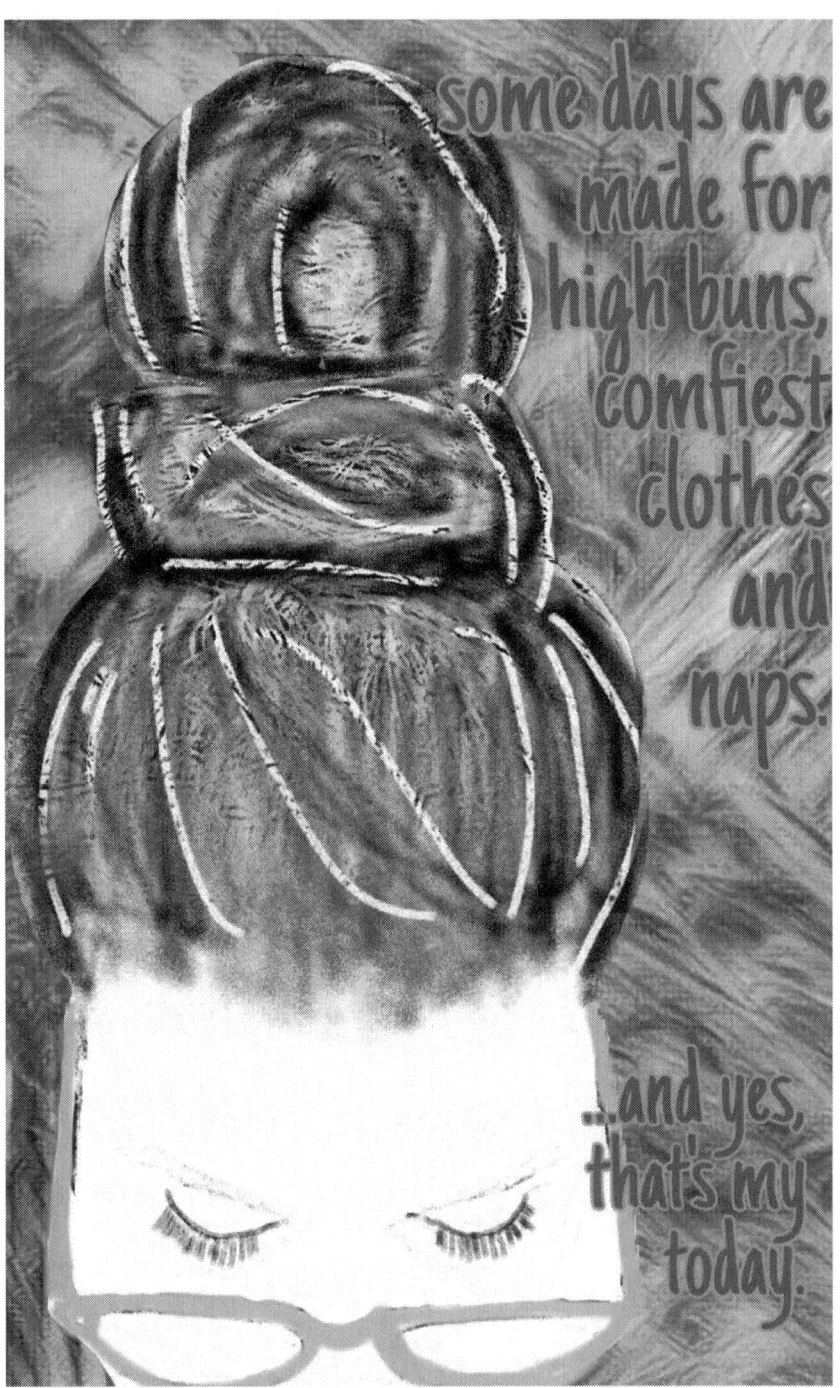

AFFIRMATION-A-DAY WITH @ME_CHRONICALLY

I am
divine
connected
expressive
loved
strong
creative
safe

Stephanie Sauer

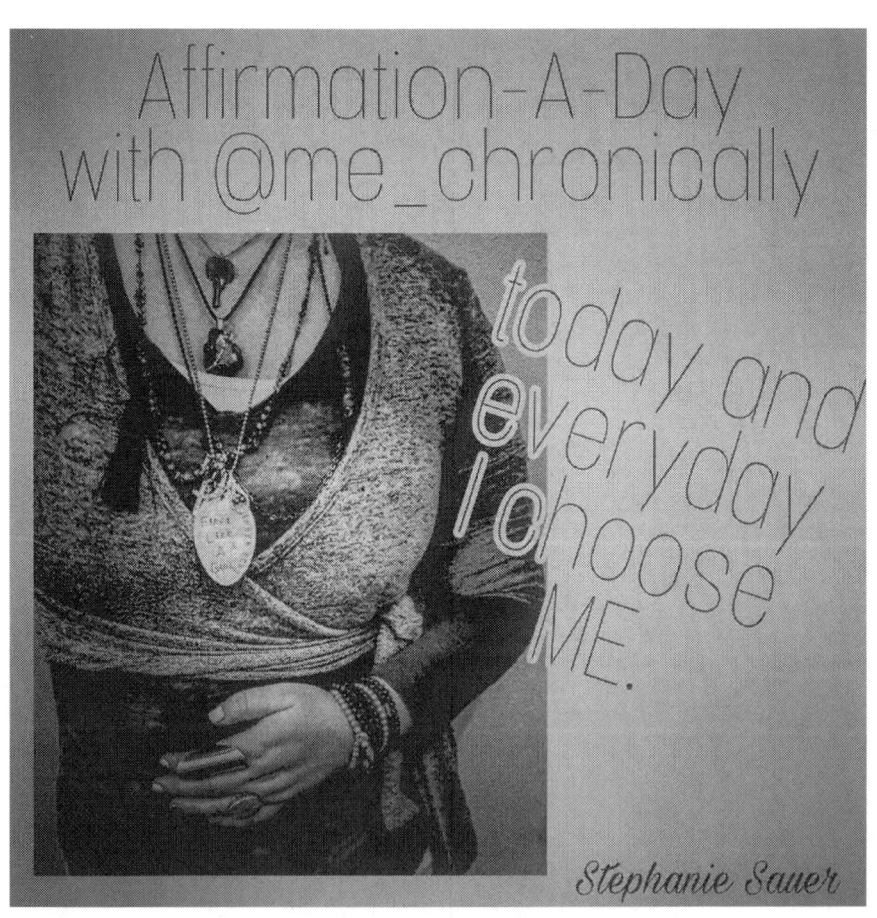

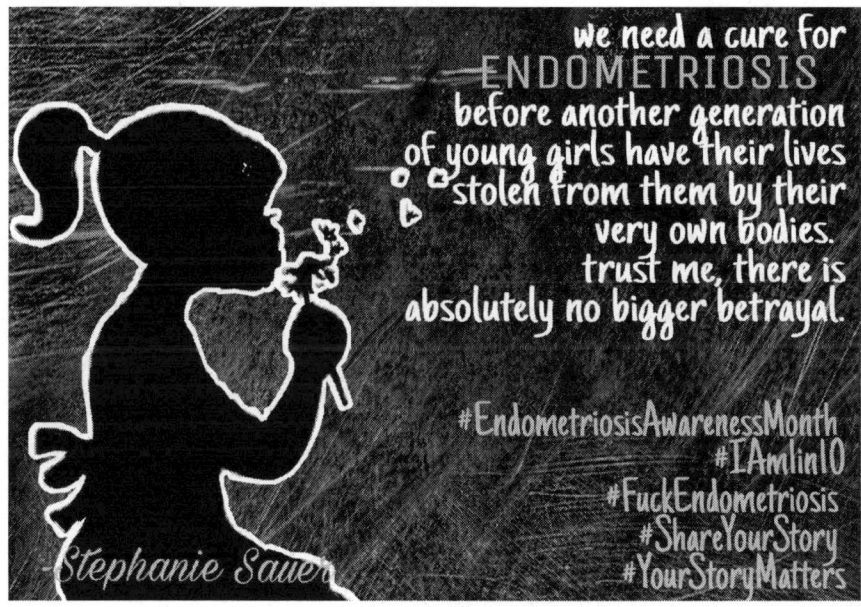

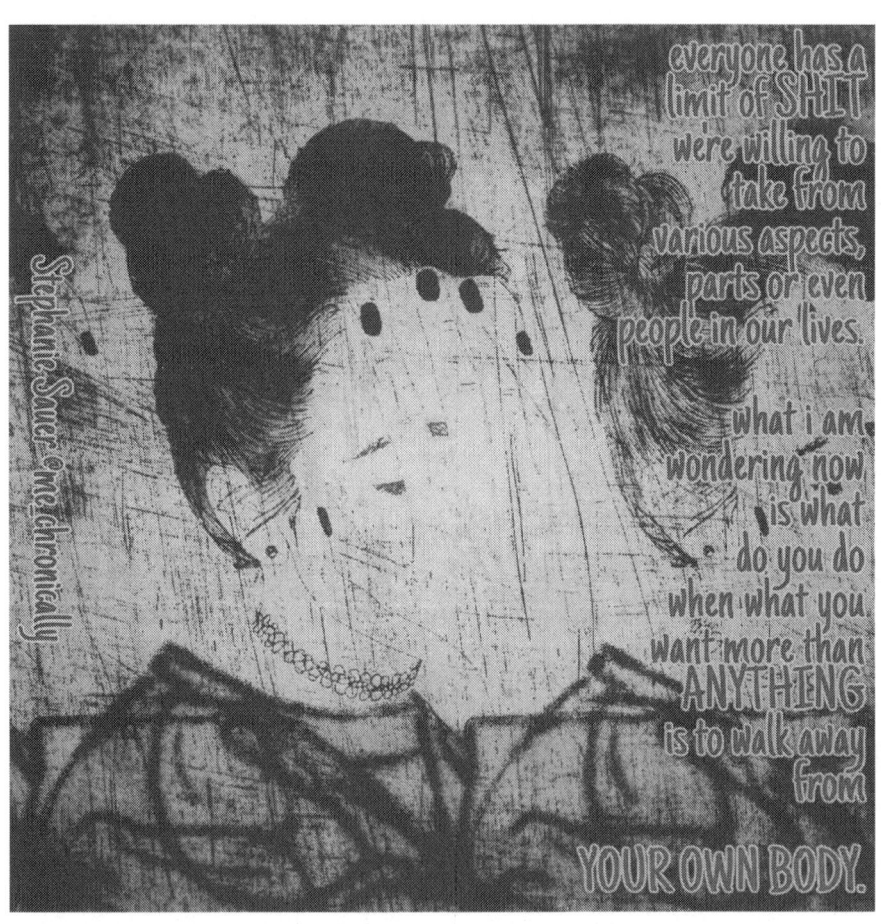

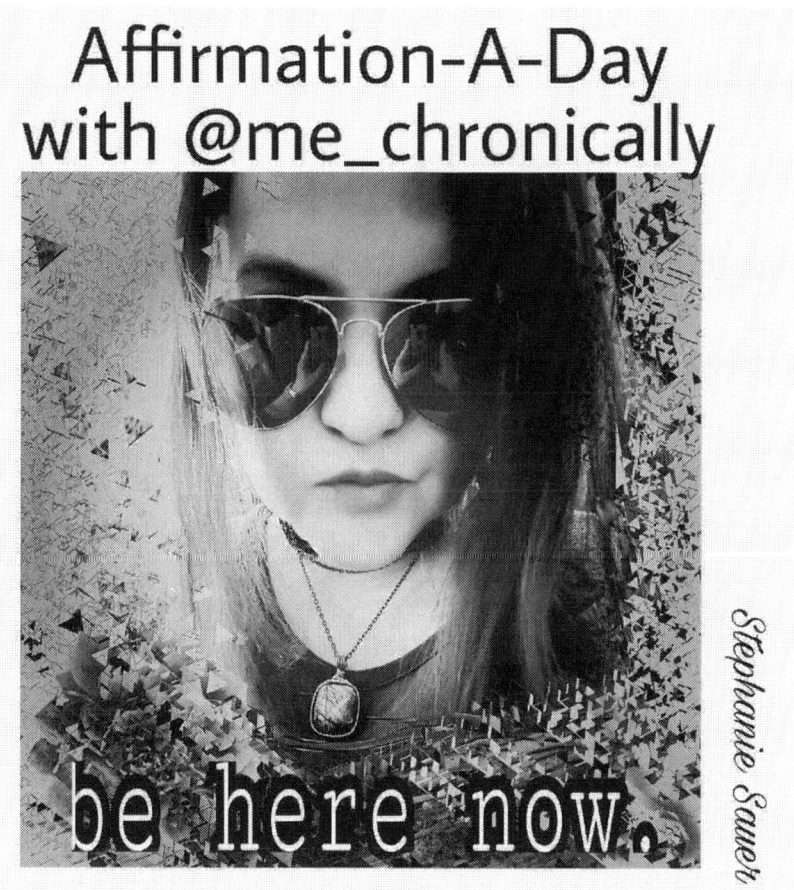

Follow me on IG @me chronically

Peace & Love,

Stephanie

> "Giving up is NOT an option."
>
> – Katrina Alleyne
> #iamanendolioness

TEN

Katrina Alleyne, Barbados

Living in Barbados, Katrina was 29 years old when she was diagnosed with Endometriosis. Today she's 34 and shares her journey with us.

Life started out normal like any teenager, but it soon came to an abrupt halt when I started to mature. The pain associated with my period was terrifying on the onset of my menstruation. As I grew older, the pain got worse and from age thirteen to age eighteen I was hospitalized for a low blood count due to the amount of blood I had lost. It was terrifying.

I grew up with the taboo stigma attached to periods and experiencing excruciating pain. I could not go to school or participate in any activities and had to take that week off from work monthly.

In 2012, the pain was at its peak, it was unimaginable. I remember it like yesterday. Having being hospitalized twice for a ruptured ovarian cyst, treated, I was sent home not knowing I would return two months after the last discharge. On my outpatient visit I was in crippling pain to the point where I couldn't walk and the doctor at the time who was my physician, Dr. Chatranni, decided that a laparoscopy was needed because of the severity of the agony that I was experiencing.

When I came back from surgery the next day they came to my bedside to break the news of their findings. My world would change for the worse, because I was diagnosed with endometriosis, a disease with no cure and pain for life was a guarantee.

I cried, I couldn't cope.

It was the first time I had heard of it. It took me twenty years to find out what was causing so much havoc in this body of mine. Now I understood I had adhesions fusing my organs together.

In 2013, I had a DNC to see if that would stop the bleeding as I was losing so much blood and had also become anemic. It didn't work.

In 2014, under the team of Dr. Chase and Dr. Bayo, I had a surgery done that brought me some temporary comfort. It didn't make sense to remove my reproductive organs, as the endometriosis had spread to various parts of my body, including my bowels and urinary tract.

I live daily with pain, but I also learn to fight when I want to give up most. People don't understand how I do it most days, especially the ones close to me. Friends on the outside looking in only see a smile, but behind closed doors are the tears and the grimacing and the many hospitalizations.

Most of all the I long for a cure, to relive life physically without pain, and follow the many career opportunities I had to put aside because of the impact this disease has had.

In 2016, after meeting so many women with the condition during hospitalizations and the passion to get the public in-the-know, I created the Katrina Endometriosis Fund Association of Barbados (registered charity #1281). It became my focus to help teenagers and women with this dreadful condition. Since then, we've done a great job getting them educated and raising awareness in the general public because even though we have a small country, many people are not aware of the condition.

My passion is to bring about sensitization to endometriosis and being the ambassador for Barbados is a privilege, because I can speak out for other women who are afraid to speak about their journey because of the stigma associated with endometriosis. The infinite fight is far from over in my ongoing journey with endometriosis, but giving up is not an option #iamanendolioness.

Words of Advice: Endometriosis is our weakness, but let our weakness become our strength.

Please connect with us on social media at Katrina Endometriosis Fund Association.

Yours Truly,
Katrina Alleyne: Endolioness

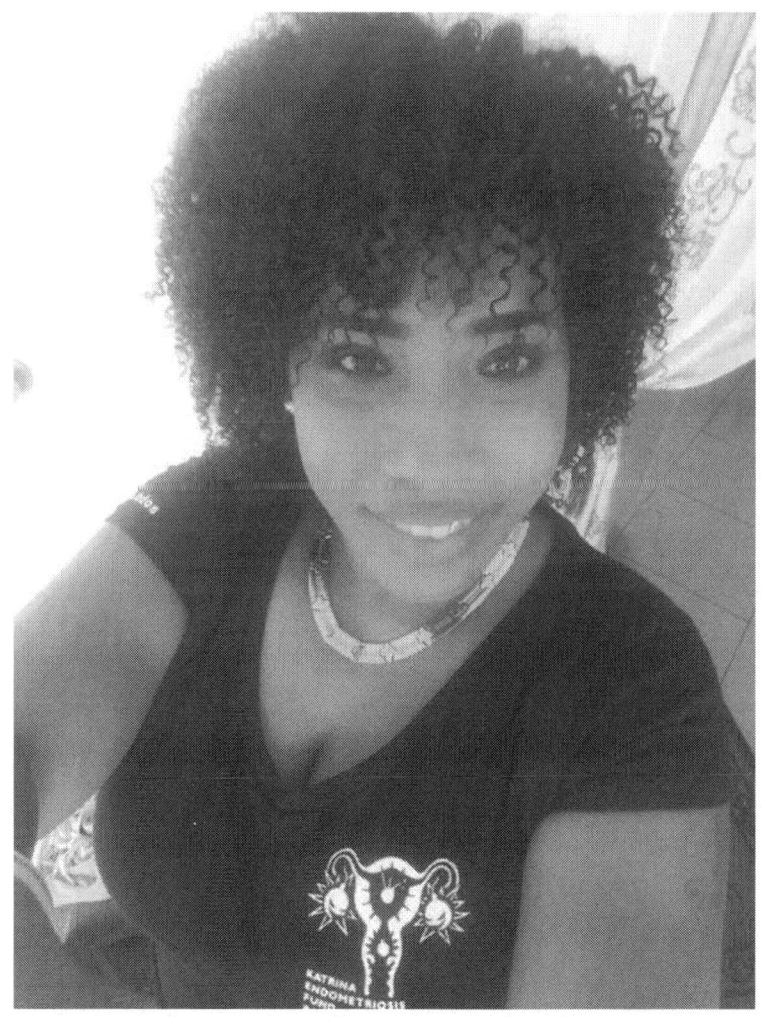

> "Endometriosis has affected and shaped every aspect of my life. I have cried oceans because of the physical and emotional pain. I have felt guilt ridden towards my family for how I isolated myself while battling this disease. I have felt shame because of work commitments I could not keep and over the years I have endlessly doubted my abilities."
>
> — Silja Steinunnardóttir

ELEVEN

Silja Steinunnardottir, Iceland

CEO The Endometriosis Association of Iceland

Hysteric Women Unite

A test of resiliance.

I wake up with searing pain. I reach out for my painkillers and swallow two parkodine forte and two ibufen. I know it won't ease the pain but it dulls my senses a little and that alone is better than nothing. I put on my heating pads which offer some relief.

As the morning continues the constant pain has me crying and moaning. I wait as long as I can to go to the bathroom but in the end I can not ignore the pressure. When I pee the pain is searing. The pressure to release stools is so urgent, yet it hurts so much to do so. I feel I am about to faint and let myself slide to the floor. When I regain consciousness the pain is unbearable. I lie on my side on the cold tiles of the bathroom floor and throw up. When the worst of the worst has passed I somehow manage to make it back to bed again.

Regardless of what my gynecologist has said, this can not be normal. I decide to call for a physician, who after some hesitation decides to call for an ambulance to take me to the hospital. When at the hospital, the pace seems slow. My blood pressure is measured, a blood sample taken and I am given one meager panodil for my pain. As the day goes by, my pain slowly becomes more bearable. I am utterly exhausted and nod on and off to sleep. Finally I am told, they can find nothing wrong with me and it is agreed that I can go for a check up at the Department of Obstertics and Gynaecology. When there, the sonar examination shows nothing as usual and I am sent home without any recomendations.

During my next acute pain attack I am going to stay at home and not spend my precious energy on a pointless hospital visit. Sometimes I wish I would just die. Not because I have a tendancy towards depression but because the constant pain and everything it entails is so bad that it's unberable to live with.

The Endometriosis journey
I was diagnosed with endometriosis at the age of 28 in the year 1999. The description above is the combined story of two trips I made to the emergency room around that time. I never did go there again. It felt so pointless. The laparatomy in which I received diagnosis, only offered temporary relief and I was given little follow up treatment or information about the disease. Therefor I soon afterwards found myself back in the horrible reality of extreme pain and exhaustion. I also felt more hopeless than ever since the surgery and diagnosis did not offer the cure I had, in my ignorance, believed it would do. It was not until in my mid thirties when I started educating myself about endometriosis and found Iceland's leading specialist in endometriosis, that I slowly began to reclaim my health.

Endometriosis has been a big part of my life journey. It has has affected and shaped every aspect of my life. I have cried oceans because of the physical and emotional pain which endometriosis entails. I have felt guilt ridden towards my family for how I isolated myself while battling this disease. I have felt shame because of work commitments I could not keep and over the years I have endlessly doubted my abilities. Two laparatomies, three laparascopies, three failed IVU's, and one gastroscopy are merely landmarks on a road filled with pain and grief. Because of endometriosis, I quit high school, worked part time for many years, had lower income and slower progress on the labour market than I otherwise would have had. Endometriosis put a strain on my relationship with my ex partner and because of endometriosis I lost contact with friends, had few moments with my family and had great difficulty starting a family of my own.

Finding a good phycisian – your life's lottery prize
Although healthcare provided for women with endometriosis in Iceland has improved since I faced my worst battles, the changes are surprisingly

insignificant. In Iceland, as elsewhere, we have a long way to go concerning diagnosis and healthcare provided for women with endometriosis.

A woman might first seek the help of the family doctor who in some cases points her to a gynecologist but might just as well only offer her painkillers with the message that this is simply a woman's lot in life. When she does get an appointment with a gynecologist it is also uncertain where that will lead.

Therefore, when a woman with endometriosis seeks help, one could compare it to buying a lottery ticket. Will she be lucky? Will she receive diagnosis early on, proper follow up treatment and therefore have a chance of a life of opportunities instead of obstacles or will she thread the begging route between specialists for years, without being diagnosed? Will she be given the impression, her problems are mainly in her head or worse yet, go through multiple laparoscopys where only a small portion of her disease is excised?

It is a grave matter, that the quality of a person's life, who seeks help because of a serious disease, is so dependent on happenstance. Let me give you some examples.

Five days diagnosis time
If there is such a thing as a positive endometriosis story, my friend Sóldís's would be it. Sóldís Lilja Benjamínsdóttir is a 35 years old physiotherapy student at the University of Iceland. She started her period at age 16. She experienced bad pain from the start but it was usually managable with painkillers. At age 31 she experienced her first acute pain attack. She sought help on Tuesday and on Friday she had a laparascopy and was diagnosed with endometriosis. Although I know of women who "only" had a diagnosis delay of a few years, I have never heard of such a quick process as was the case with Sóldís. To quote Sóldís:

"My doctor has been very helpful. She answered my questions and her treatment has proven successful. The Endometriosis Association suggested her to me. It was good to be able to contact them and get advice which proved to be so helpful."

27 years diagnosis time

Ragnheiður's story is quite a different one. Ragnheiður K. Jóhannesdóttir Thoroddsen is 47 years old and has a B.Sc. in tourism studies and business management.

Ragnheiður started her period at age thirteen and experienced severe pain from the start. At fourteen she sought help for the first time and was given painkillers. Following that she went between gyneocologists and other specialists almost on a yearly basis and not one of them mentioned the possibility of endometriosis. Through her teenage years and adulthood she dug deep to get through life. She repeatedly overdid herself, which took its toll.

Eventually, during internet research, she stumbled upon the web page of The Endometrioisis Association of Iceland and realized she had all the listed symptoms except infertility. This led to her diagnosis of endometriosis in 2012, 27 years after her symptoms started and 26 years after she first sought help because of them.

Ragnheiður has since then, had a hysterectomy and been diagnosed with fybromalgia. On top of that, in 2017, a tumor in her colon was detected which doctors believed to be cancerous. Ragnheiður herself was of the opinion that the tumor was endometriosis and on her request, an endometriosis surgeon took part in a surgery where the tumor was removed along with a part of her colon. As Ragnheiður had anticipated, the tumor turned out to be endometriosis. Today, pain is still a part of her everyday life. To quote Ragnheiður

"It´s much too exspensive for society to judge women by their looks! Endometriosis is real and needs to be treated, to prevent women from developing fatigue, infertility etc."

Ragnheiður had been lucky enough to bear two children. In her opinion her illness has affected them and their life as a family tremendously. This former business woman, has been on disability benefits since 2013. One cannot but wonder, how different her life might have been, if she had undergone surgery and received diagnosis earlier, followed with the needed healthcare. Which leads us to our young ones.

A very severe case of "exam anxiety"
Hafdís Houmøller Einarsdóttir started having her period at age twelve which from the beginning was very painful. During her worst accute pain attacks she was repeatedly taken to hospital by ambulance. But because Hafdís was under the age of eighteen she was always taken to the Children's Hospital, where no gyneocologist was called for. Finally, three years ago, at the age of eighteen, Hafdís found an endometriosis specialist and had a laparascopy where endometrosis was confirmed. To quote Hafdís:

"I realised there was no place for me in the healthcare system. What do you do with a seventeen year old, lying on the floor unable to cry because the pain is so unbearable?"

Margrét Finney Jónsdóttir is twenty one years old and shares a similar story to Hafdís. As a teenager she was repeatedly taken to the Children's Hospital during her acute pain attacks. Through another route she eventually was able to have a laparascopy and was diagnosed with endometriosis shortly before her eighteenth birthday. To quote Margrét Finney:

"One time, at The Children's Hospital, I had been given morphine throughout the night. I had vomited repeatedly and experienced the worst pain I could ever imagine. In the morning the doctors said they thought the pain could be attributed to exam anxiety. It's not that they don't want to help, it just seems as if they don't have the necessary knowledge."

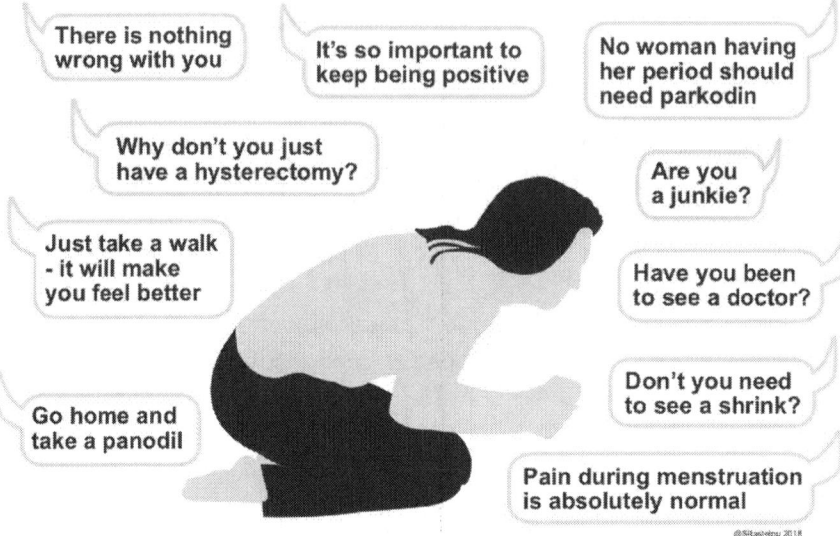

The stereotypical hysterical woman

This lack of awareness about endometriosis leads to a reality like the one portraid in the photo above. It shows direct quotes – words spoken to women with endometriosis by their family, friends, coworkers and physicians. Words which shed a light on how often the pain of women with endometriosis is deemed insignificant. Words which show that the idea of the stereotypical hysteric woman seems to be well and alive today, however unaware people are of it.

The Emergency Room is no exception. Luck could be with you. But it could just as well not be. As was the case with one of our endo sisters, who at the start of her period went to the ER on a regular basis but staff never mentioned the possibility of endometriosis. To quote a Member of the Endometriosis Association of Iceland in 2012:

"It's bewildering that one can go to the emergency room every month, with abdominal pain, always at the start of menstruation – and doctor's don't put two and two together. I can't have been the only woman who has sought their help because of pain which is so bad she can neither sit nor stand."

I would like to mention that of course everything is not as bad as all that. I love my endometriosis surgeon dearly and I have deep regard for our healthcare professionals who work under more straining conditions than I can probably ever imagine. Yet these stories of long diagnosis time and inadequate healthcare highlight that there is certainly room for improvement within the healthcare system. Surely these women deserve better.

Gender bias within the healthcare system
Research from 2008 shows that women in USA nationwide, wait on average for 65 minutes before receiving an analgesic at the ER for acute abdominal pain. Men on the other hand, wait an average of 49 minutes for the same service.

Literature seems to support the assumption that there is a gender bias regarding women's pain experiences. For instance, a study in 2014 at the Sahlgrenska University Hospital in Sweden, showed that female patients generally waited longer than male patients at the emergency department and male patients were more often given a higher prioritized color in the triage process.

One cannot but wonder why, in the year 2019, we are still here? Why is the pain of women not taken more seriously? Why is there not more awareness about endometriosis, a disease which symptoms have been known for centuries?

Colossal mass misdiagnosis
The Nezhat brothers, the well known gynecological surgeons and their team, took to history books to recover information about endometriosis through the centuries. They are of the opinion that many of the women, Dr. Freud "diagnosed" as hysterical in his time, did in fact have endometriosis. Their overall conclusion was that the treatment of women with endometriosis through the ages constituted one of the most colossal mass misdiagnoses in human history, one that over the centuries has subjected women to murder, madhouses and lives of unremitting physical, social, and psychological pain.

Perhaps we should pause a while to let that sink in. This in a way, is the heritage we are still dealing with.

Endometriosis – a feminist issue?

Nancy Petersen is a nurse who has been a long time advocate for endometriosis awareness and as such is a legend in her own right. To quote Nancy:

"If 176 million men had endometriosis it would be an international emergency. We would not let a disease destroy their lives, their careers, their sexuality, their fertility, their joy in life for a minute. And we would not dismiss them as neurotic."

I cannot but agree. The pain of endometriosis alone is often traumatic. Not being believed about said pain is surely traumatising. Because our pain is not taken seriously enough, we women may need to express ourselves more strongly to be heard. But then if we do, we run the risk of being labeled neurotic. The irony is that with long diagnosis time, dismissal of symptoms, suggestions of hysteria on top of dealing with a difficult disease, we women with endometriosis do have a strong reason to become, dare I say it, hysterical!

Our time has come

In December 2017, the minister of health in Australia, Greg Hunt announced he was setting up a national action plan to improve treatment of women with endometriosis and that research funding for endometriosis would be increased. Hunt also apologised to women with endometriosis that nothing had been done sooner.

To me these news from the other side of the world, seemed quite a milestone on a long and difficult journey. It is time that societies and officials openly admit that women with endometriosis have been wronged. It is time that calculated, informed actions are taken to correct that wrongdoing. It is time that the neccesary steps are taken to ensure women with endometriosis receive the healthcare they deserve and need.

Endometriosis is a serious disease which can have serious repercussions. It does not just affect the reproductive organs but can impact many other organs and in fact almost all parts of the body. Endometriosis is complex and calls for a multidisciplinary approach, a team of specialists in different fields and experienced excision surgeons.

Educating oneself about endometriosis can seem like an overwhelming burden when all one's willpower is needed just to get through the day. Yet I urge you, women with endometriosis, to do so.

Women with endometriosis, reach out to others who share your experiences. Speak up, share your stories, do your research, advocate for yourselves, ask difficult questions, press for better healthcare. Our time has come! Let's get our revolution going. "Hysteric" women unite!

This article is partly based on an article by the author which was published in Fréttablaðið newspaper and on www.visir.is on February 23, 2012 and partly on her lecture at the AAGL Global Endometriosis Summit in Harpa, Reykjavík, Iceland, July 20-21, 2017.

Silja Steinunnardóttir (@siljasteinu) is CEO of The Endometriosis Association of Iceland. Earlier she was chairman of the board for six years. In cooperation with the association's board, she organized the first endometriosis conference in Iceland in 2012, Iceland's participation in the Million Women March for Endometriosis 2014, the association's ten year's anniversary event in 2016, a forum about endometriosis in 2017, a forum about endometriosis in teens in 2018 as well as the association's yearly awareness week and participation in the Reykjavík marathon. As chairman, she has emphasized raising awareness about endometriosis. She has pushed for a multi-disciplinary approach to treating women with endometriosis and the establishing of a formal endometriosis center in Iceland. Silja strives for the association's main objective, which is to assist women with endometriosis. Silja has published numerous articles about endometriosis in Icelandic media and been interviewed repeatedly on the subject. She did a lecture at the AAGL Global Endometriosis Summit, in Reykjavík Iceland 2017 and at the 5th Nordic Conference on Endometriosis, in Odense Denmark in 2018.

The Endometriosis Association of Iceland (@endoiceland) was founded in 2006 and is a non profit organisation. Its main objective is to assist women with endometriosis and their families. The association also advocates for the establishment of an endometriosis center in Iceland and a multi disciplinary approach to the treatment of women with endometriosis. It has been fundamental in raising awareness about endometriosis in Iceland and has thus been crucial in giving Icelandic women with endometriosis a voice.

References

Camran Nezhat, M.D., Farr Nezhat, M.D., and Ceana Nezhat, M.D., Endometriosis: ancient disease, ancient treatments, Fertility and Sterility, 2012, vol. 98, page 1.

Chen EH et al., Gender disparity in analgesic treatment of emergency department patients with acute abdominal pain, Academic Emergency Treatment, 2008.

Diane E. Hoffmann and Anita J. Tarzian, The Girl Who Cried Pain: A Bias Against Women in the Treatment of Pain, Journal of Law, Medicine & Ethics, 2001, vol. 29, page 21.

Gabrielle Jackson, Greg Hunt apologises to women with endometriosis and announces action plan, Guardian, December, 2017.

Joe Fassler, How Doctors Take Women's Pain Less Seriously, The Atlantic, 2015.

Josefina Robertson, Waiting Time at the Emergency Department from a Gender Equality Perspective, Master Thesis in Medicine, Institute of Medicine at the Sahlgrenska Academy University of Gothenburg, 2014.

Kayla Webley Adler, Women are dying because doctors treat us like men, Marie Claire, May, 2017.

Nancy Petersen, If 176 million men had endometriosis, LinkedIn, 2015.

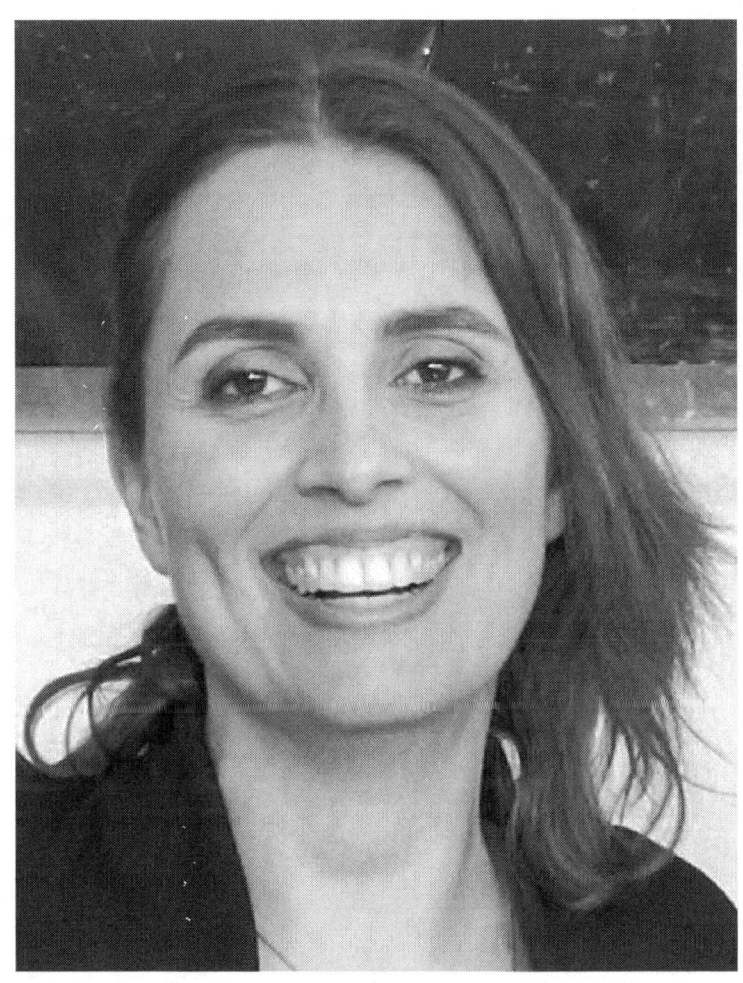

Pictured: Silja Steinunnardóttir

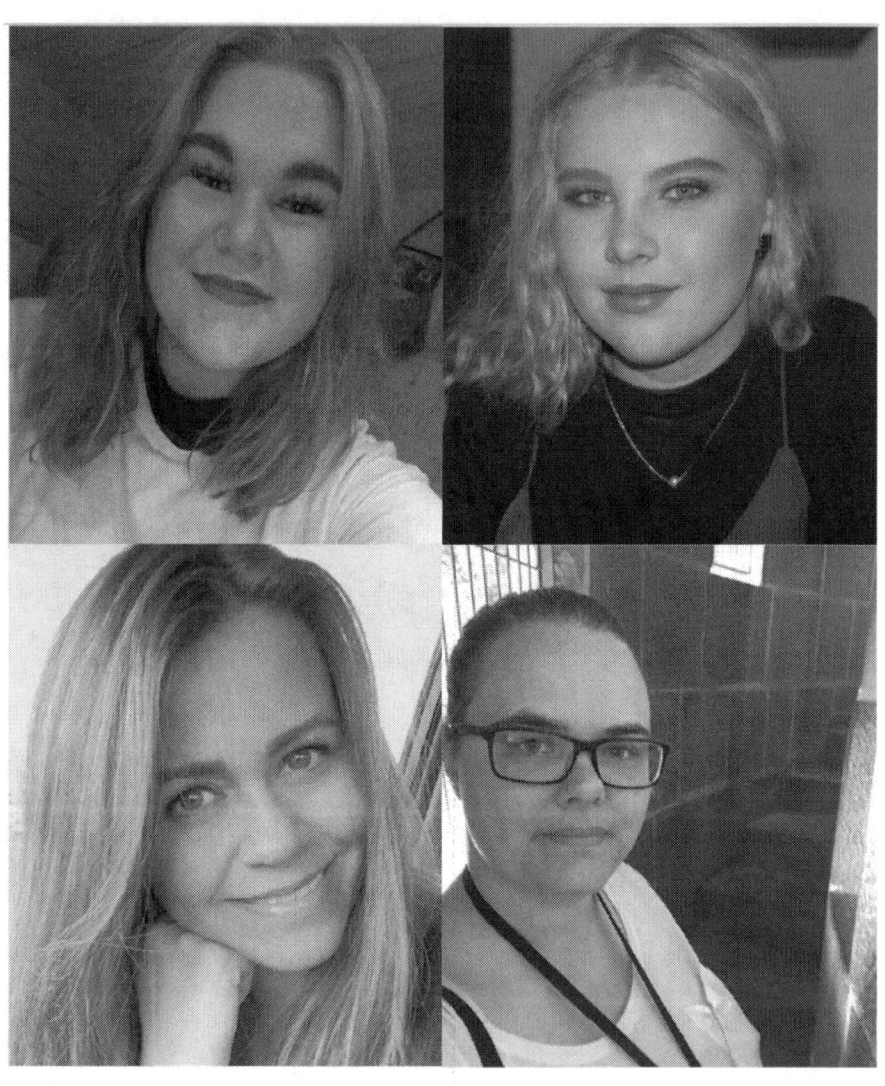

Pictured clockwise from top left:
Margrét Finney Jónsdóttir
Hafdís Houmøller Einarsdóttir
Ragnheiður K. Jóhannesdóttir Thoroddsen
Sóldís Lilja Benjamínsdóttir

> "I've been to at least 20 doctors trying to find answers. I've had my appendix, gallbladder, ovaries, uterus, and cervix removed ... all by different doctors, because after surgery they would tell me there was nothing else they could do for me, even though I was still in pain."
>
> — Samantha Bowick

TWELVE

Samantha Bowick, South Carolina

A Life Interrupted by Endometriosis
Samantha Bowick, MPH, 28 years old

I started my period when I was in 8th grade. I always had heavy periods and severe cramping that would leave me missing school and later college classes.

When I was about 16 years old, I went to my first gynecologist and told her about my symptoms. She suggested that I try birth control pills to help make my periods regular and decrease the pain that I was having every month.

I graduated high school with a high GPA, despite my pain and went on to attend college in my hometown. During high school, I worked up front at a pharmacy and transferred over to the pharmacy side and became a pharmacy technician once I graduated high school. I just knew I wanted to be a pharmacist.

During my second semester of college is when my pain became unbearable. I noticed my pain was occurring more frequently and went back to my gynecologist. We talked about laparoscopic surgery in the middle of 2010 and decided to do my first one in the following weeks. I was 19.

During the surgery my gynecologist found that I had endometriosis, which she cauterized. However, there was some disease she did not remove because she said it was too close to my ovaries.

A few weeks after surgery, I was still having pain. She said that I should not be in as much pain and that there was nothing else I could do.

There were so many nights that I was unable to sleep, because I was in so much pain and in tears. The nausea, debilitating pain, and heavy periods were awful to deal with. I just wanted a doctor who would listen and help me.

Since then, I have had five additional surgeries from 2012-2016, which have resulted in endometriosis being cauterized and excised; removal of my appendix, gallbladder, both ovaries, uterus, and cervix; and many abdominal scars. All of these were done by different doctors because after I had a surgery with one, they would tell me there was nothing else they could do for me, even though I was still in pain.

I have been to at least 20 doctors trying to find answers for my pain and symptoms. This has been a financial drain on me and my family, even when I had medical insurance.

I had plans to attend pharmacy school, but that changed when my pain continued after each surgery (except for my last one) and other health issues that I have had. I was accepted to pharmacy school twice, but withdrew from the programs because of my health. I have attended college online and received my Bachelor of Science in Health Care Administration from Columbia Southern University in 2014 and Master of Public Health from Liberty University in 2017.

I have also been diagnosed with vitamin D deficiency, irritable bowel syndrome, interstitial cystitis, osteoporosis, polycystic ovary syndrome, and retroperitoneal fibrosis during one of my surgeries. I have been to doctors in South Carolina, Georgia, and Florida trying to find answers for endometriosis.

It has been difficult for me not to isolate myself, because of the pain I have experienced over the years, not being able to have kids, and dealing with other health issues. Over the years, I have had to cancel plans and stop doing things that most people my age do, which has resulted in me losing friends along the way.

However, I am fortunate to have my family and friends who have remained in my life and support me throughout all of this and I am very thankful for them. My faith has kept me strong in the fight against endometriosis.

I started writing Living with Endometriosis: The Complete Guide to Risk Factors, Symptoms, and Treatment Options in 2013, while I was attending pelvic floor physical therapy. I want to help other women who suffer with endometriosis get the answers they need for their pain and symptoms and to know they are not alone.

In this book, I detail what treatments I have tried, the surgeries I have had, the doctors I have been to, as well as medical research and information about endometriosis. Writing also helped me release many negative emotions that I have had with endometriosis and the changes it has brought to my life.

I will never get pregnant and have children "naturally," as I had a hysterectomy at 23 years old. At the time I felt this is what I needed to do to get out of pain since I had tried several birth controls, Lupron (which caused horrible side effects), diet changes, pelvic floor physical therapy, exercises, supplements, bioidentical hormones, and surgery (but not with an endometriosis specialist until after my hysterectomy). MRIs, CT scans, and colonoscopies were done, but always came back normal.

It is awful that many doctors do not know enough about endometriosis and we are left to find answers for ourselves and do our own research. It is important that we are our own health advocate and do not agree to anything we do not want to.

Unfortunately, this is the reality for at least 176 million women worldwide and is a serious public health issue. It is heartbreaking that many of us are unable to work, especially when we want to, but cannot because of our health.

It is devastating the number of women who commit suicide because they are in so much pain, cannot find the answers they need, and feel like their pain is all in their head.

There is a community of us trying to bring more awareness to the disease so that more research will be done to find more answers that will benefit all of us who suffer with endometriosis. We need treatment options that are less invasive and more practical for our bodies; we need a cure.

Keep telling your stories and keep fighting.

If you are interested in learning more about my story, *Living with Endometriosis: The Complete Guide to Risk Factors, Symptoms and Treatment Options.*

Website: https://www.samanthabowick.com

Samantha Bowick, MPH, BSHCA

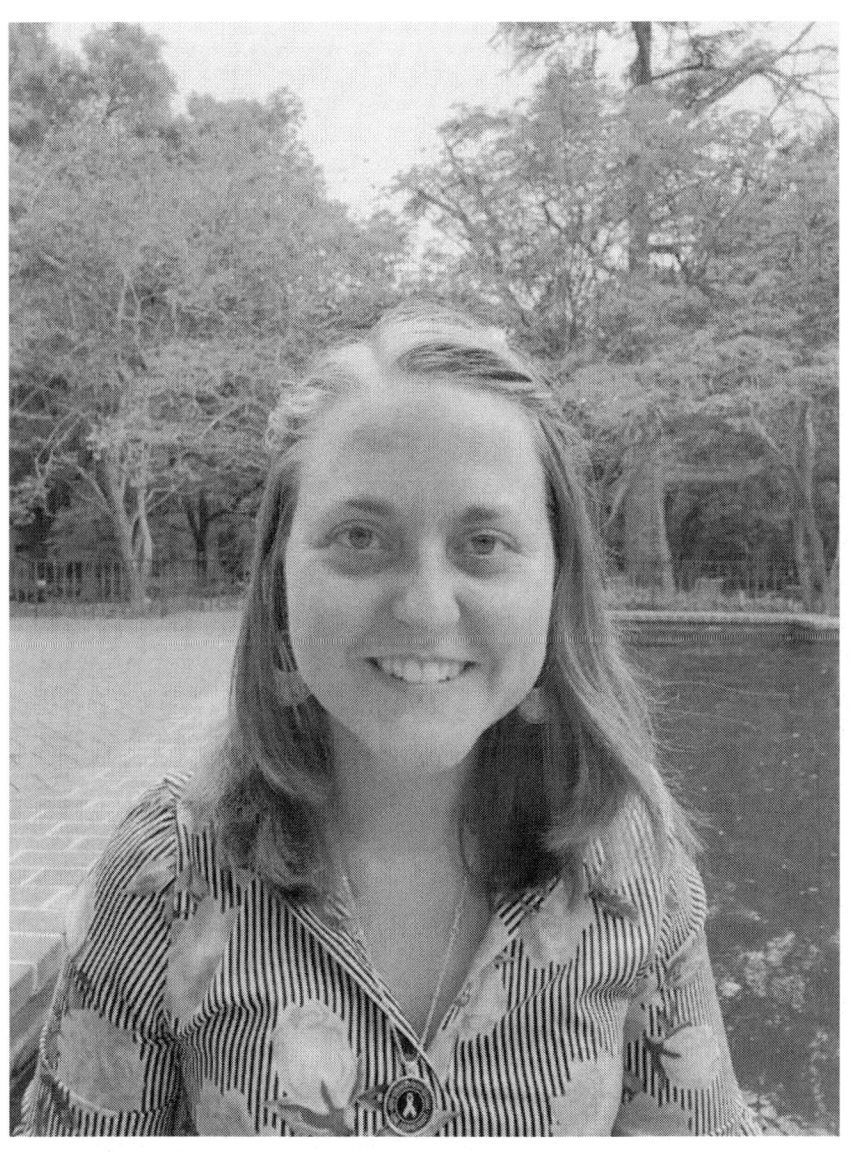

"My favorite leggings went into the garbage that day. They were only the first of many articles of clothing I would bleed through. Despite ample protection during my cycle I frequently bled too heavily. Each time I ruined something my parents yelled. More than twenty years later we would learn that heavy cycle wasn't actually my fault."

— Dr. Sallie Sarrel, PT ATC DPT

THIRTEEN

Dr. Sallie Sarrel, PT ATC DPT, East Coast

My Cotton Club

My best friend still didn't need to wear a bra. She was fifteen. Her body was straight in what I thought were all the right places. She got her first period when she was away at camp. These were the days before cell phones. She waited all day to be allowed to use the telephone open to campers for special occasions like birthdays, anniversaries and apparently your first menses. She was exuberant on the phone as she told her mother and her mother was almost crying happy tears.

A few days later a package arrived at camp for my friend. She grabbed at its contents. Her aunt had made a rose bouquet out of tampons with attached a note, "Welcome to the cotton club" That string and cotton bouquet is still displayed in her home all these years later.

Stark contrast from my first period. I was just thirteen. My cousins and I were playing card games underneath the table at the Spanish restaurant where we were celebrating my grandmother's 80th birthday. In true 1980's style, I was wearing leggings and an oversized button down with a long necklace of fake pearls knotted in the middle. I was curvy. This outfit was my favorite.

I was difficult to fit—a just out of sixth grade girl with a D-sized chest. This outfit camouflaged everything while still being the height of teen style. I noticed the blood stains in my clothes before I left the restaurant, yet I said nothing until the next morning when I realized someone was going to have to go to the drugstore.

I was ashamed of it right from the start. At school the girls my age who had their periods were the overweight girls no one wanted to be friends with.

They had pain, missed school or sat in the nurse's office during gym. All of a sudden, by some crazy twist of fate called hormones, this life was upon me.

I must have sat on the toilet for twenty minutes crying before I called for help from my mother. It's hard to imagine that on some level my 13 year old self knew my life was damaged forever. My mother groaned when I told her. She had gone into menopause when I was 5 years old, when she was 36. We had nothing in the house but the sample sanitary napkin my school had sent home when they explained puberty to the students. My feelings or need for privacy were not even considered. I was mortified when she told my father.

This was endometriosis, except I would not know the indelible mark the disease made until I was diagnosed 25 years later.

My favorite leggings went into the garbage that day. They were only the first of many articles of clothing I would bleed through. Despite ample protection during my cycle I frequently bled too heavily. Each time I ruined something my parents yelled. More than twenty years later we would learn that heavy cycle wasn't actually my fault.

I was nearly 35 when I was diagnosed with endometriosis, a disease in which tissue similar to but not the same as the lining of the uterus wrecks havoc on your abdomen, pelvis and back or more. Even a diagnosis doesn't take the sting out of just how many outfits I lost. Secretly I stayed up late, wrestling back pain and intense cramping, to rinse clothes out while everyone slept. I learned to hide. I hid – hid my pain, hid the monthly ordeal.

When my first period arrived there was no way to tell all those years ago that something inside would go terribly haywire causing my pelvic organs to adhere to themselves. But, yet the doom and gloom I felt that first morning calling for my mother, I feel each and every cycle. I'll have approximately 470 cycles in a lifetime. Never once have I been filled with the excitement my friend felt that day at camp.

As an teen with undiagnosed endometriosis, the cotton club was just about the most horrible place to be. Getting up to go to school with horrible cramps or using super-sized tampons as 14 year old in an effort to prevent mishaps was unpleasant to say the least.

As I got into high school I would rise extra early to combat the stomach issues I had with my cycle and still make it to school on time. As an adult I've missed work, social enjoyments and all sorts of possibilities because of anguish.

By 36, not a single egg was left in my body. I battled and paid for six surgeries, not to mention modified diets, years of physical therapy and a longing in my heart just to be a more "normal" woman. Until diagnosis, I did not know sex wasn't supposed to hurt and I am a pelvic health specialist.

My cotton club has brought me years of pain and agony. My cotton club has given me scars both physical and emotional. My cotton club never included a new mommy club. I never went to this club in white shorts while skipping in a field the way the TV commercials depict a period. There are days when I feel hopeless, there are days when I feel as if I can't take it anymore.

Years ago, my favorite 12 year old, who happens to have cerebral palsy, asked me to lunch. She had something to discuss with me, something she did not want to talk about with her mother. She seemed so happy and so innocent when she quietly turned to me and asked, "What's it like to have your period?"

Uncharacteristically I stepped out of my practitioner role and without hesitation leaned forward," Having your period is by far the worst thing that ever happens to you and it happens once a month." She sunk into her chair, suddenly small and disappointed. My little buddy was already scared of the changes in her body. I was making all those fears come true. I turned to her," I have a disease that makes my periods worse. I don't just get my period I spend days trying to figure out how to live through it."

She looked at me with compassion, surprising since she herself was in a wheelchair. I felt guilty for allowing her to see that I am controlled by my cycle. I forgot that getting your period for the first time signals a time of great change in a young girl's life – an exciting time that most people embrace. I spent the majority of my career since that day making sure no other teen lives the life I have had. It's been a labor of love, marred by pain and trauma. Some days I think we make a difference and some days I think the world still has no clue what endometriosis is.

What I do know is that nearly nine months later my buddy opened a package from me filled with a cotton bouquet. The cycle of the cycle begins again and as women with endometriosis we are ready to educate and advocate so no one fears their Cotton Club.

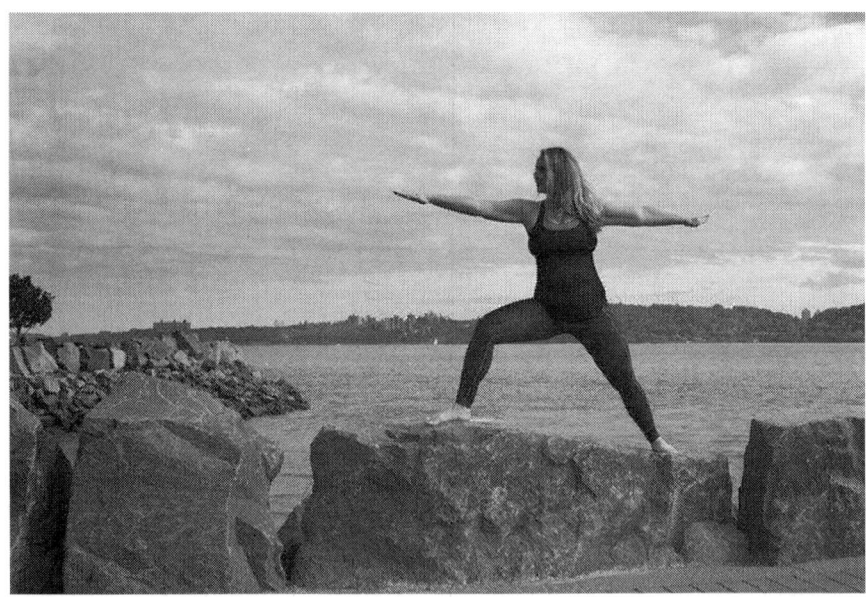

"I grew up hearing we were cursed because of Eve's decision to sin, punished into pain and childbirth."

– Lisa Howard

FOURTEEN

Lisa Howard, San Diego

My Journey

I started my period when I was 12 or 13 years old. I remember them hurting (but not as devastating as they have in my adult years), but figured it was normal.

I grew up hearing we were cursed because of Eve's decision to sin, punished into pain and childbirth. I also heard that some of my family members had really painful periods. So again, it was normal.

Classmates said they had cramps, too…so I figured mine were just normal. I became that girl in Junior High and High School that would walk around with a hoodie tied around her waist every month because I'd almost always overflow. I had classmates come up to me during the really hard cramps, ask if I was okay, because I was white as a ghost and sweating…and I'd spend time curled up in the Nurse's office after taking an Ibuprofen.

But it was normal.

Every girl went through this. Right?

My family physician had wanted me to go on birth control, but just to prevent "baby accidents" from happening, which I quickly dismissed since I had no intention of having sex. Little did I know BCP may have helped with the pain…

I became sexually active when I got married at 21 years old. Now that I'd "done the deed," I decided it was time I saw a gynecologist. My very first one. Man, was I excited. I'd discussed my painful periods and lengthy cycles, but was told nothing was abnormal.

She put me on Ortho Tri Cyclen since my husband and I didn't want children yet, in the hopes that it would regulate my cycles and pain. It did regulate the length of my cycles, but didn't help with the pain much. However, it turned me into a weight-gaining, moody, grumpy-guss. And I hated the pill.

Two years later, we decided we'd like to start our own little family, so I gladly got off the pill. The cramps were worse than before. Days of laying curled up in a ball on the bed, squeezing the hell out of my heating pad, no OTC pain meds or "specialty pills" like Midol helped – at all.

I wasn't about to exercise ("but it's so good for your period cramps," they say…you cannot get out of bed to exercise.) Didn't want sex (even though everyone says it helps with your cramps.). My bloating was so severe I'd be asked on several occasions when my baby was due. I had monthly diarrhea along with my period. It was horrible.

Our medical insurance had changed, so I found a new gynecologist. Same story: nothing abnormal about my periods.

Fast forward five years. Still not pregnant. Have done all of the homeopathic tricks in the book to conceive (including standing on my head after sex…ha!), test my fertility, monitor ovulation, etc. Neither one of us wanted IVF, so we never considered going in for any fertility tests or treatments. Every month I would start my period, every month I would be depressed at our failure.

We had friends and family who were having families of their own, I attended countless baby showers, offered way too many "congratulations." Each time, wanting to wallow in my own sadness over the fact that we have been unable to conceive. I had begun to resent those new mothers around me. At no fault of their own. I was still very happy for them…but still incredibly jealous, sad, and even angry. It was a dark and horrible downward spiral. We eventually stopped trying and hoped it would just happen on it's own.

My gynecologist had retired, so I was assigned a new one at Kaiser. At my next annual pap appointment, the new doctor agreed: nothing abnormal about my period pain or cycles. She did discover however, that I had a septated vaginal canal. A split down the center of my vagina, so that I have a right side and a left side. My right side was normal leading straight to my cervix, but the left side just dead-ended at the back of my vaginal canal. She surmised that if we had been having sex on the left side and his semen was just hitting a blocked wall, making it impossible to conceive. So we tried making sure he was on the right side during intercourse. Still no pregnancy.

Which was a good thing. In 2009, we separated. My marriage had ended. Add that to my growing emotional pit.

Since I had left my husband, I had to get my own health insurance which means, you guessed it: a new gynecologist. My first visit to this doctor was hilarious. Within seconds of descending between the cleft of my thighs, he popped his head up in excitement, "You have two!" I told him I knew I had two sides. "No," he said, "you have two cervix!"

WHAT?

How in the world did my three…THREE…prior gynecologists miss the fact that I have two fully-functioning cervix? This doctor was so excited he had to invite a few staff members and specialists in to look for themselves (with my permission, of course).

After the excitement died down, he told me that my right side was wider, but my cervical opening was tiny. My left side was much narrower, but my cervical opening was normal. He figured we hadn't been getting pregnant because of the tiny opening on the right. He also said women with "this condition" have a very hard time naturally conceiving. "Nearly impossible," he said. So I resigned myself to not having children. He also believed my period pain and cycles were "normal."

He was also the first gynecologist to prescribe me pain medication for my horrendous cramps. Naproxen Sodium. Iit was the only thing that worked. I took those pills every month until my excision surgery in 2014. Five years of having to depend on pharmaceuticals to help alleviate my pain. Sometimes they didn't work at all. Most times I had nausea, exhaustion, and dizziness from those pills. Sometimes I was afraid to drive. I nearly fell down the stairs on more than one occasion. Not an easy pill to stomach.

I had been routinely reprimanded at work for all of the time I had missed. I called in sick for one or two days every month. Sometimes three. I had exhausted my sick time and had to start using vacation time. I was told if I missed another day, "disciplinary action" would be taken. So I would go to work in pure agony.

I had cancelled dates and appointments because of my pain. But again…"it was normal." Fast forward to 2012 and I moved to San Diego. New job, clean slate (new vacation and sick time), new insurance, and yep, a new gynecologist. I told him about my septated canal, my double cervix (which lead into one uterus), but I had been told for so long that my periods were normal that I didn't bring it up. He asked if I experienced any cramps and what the length of my cycles were, which I answered. No surprise. He advised me to continue to take my Naproxen Sodium as needed, but a hysterectomy may one day cure those cramps.

In 2013, he wanted an ultrasound because I had expressed some tenderness during my pap. He discovered I had a small cyst on my right ovary. When I went in for a follow-up ultrasound, I now had a cyst on my left ovary. Every few months, we continued this little dance and watched the cysts grow, disappear, and reappear.

During all of this, my periods continued their harsh game, I continued to miss work at the new job (1-3 days a month), and it was mentioned in my review that I had been missing an awful lot of work once a month…Fuck.

Finally in 2014, an ultrasound showed a larger cyst on my left ovary. So my doctor ordered an MRI to get a better look at it. MRI results were read and they believed I had a dermoid cyst on my left ovary, which could potentially become cancerous. It looked like I also had abnormally thick uterine lining, which may have explained the cramping and lengthy periods. Due to the scary cancer possibility, we decided to do a routine robotic laparoscopy and remove the cyst. While I was under, he was going to perform a D&C procedure, where they scoop out that excess lining in my uterus (gross!).

Surgery. The last thing I remember was the anesthesiologist talking to me about my favorite hiking spots in San Diego (may I just say that's the BEST way to fall asleep?). My 1.5-hour surgery ended up being four hours.

Once he was inside, my gynecologist (he was also my surgeon! LOVE HIM!) was surprised to immediately notice the unmistakable signs of Endometriosis: implants and adhesions. What was thought to be a dermoid cyst was an endometrioma, also known as a chocolate cyst. My abdominal cavity was invaded by Endometriosis implants. My bladder was glued to my uterus by adhesions. My bowel was also stuck to my uterus. I had adhesions and implants on my liver and diaphragm, too. It is my understanding that he couldn't remove it from my liver and risk puncturing or damaging that organ, but he smeared some type of barrier medication to hopefully stop it from growing. And he managed to save my ovaries.

I have since altered my diet to a more Endo-friendly diet. I've also received six grueling months of Lupron Depot injections. And I am now on a continuous birth control pill, called Amethyst. So far I am pain-free. But…for now…pain free. I'm terrified for the day if it returns…but at least I now have the love and support I need…

Update: I had a second excision surgery in September, 2016. I also had another excision surgery in July 2018 and a bowel resection surgery for Endometriosis in November 2018.

Discovering I have Endometriosis has changed my life.

I'm horrified and saddened that none of my prior gynecologists ever suggested or hinted that I may have this very common disease. Let alone noticed I had two sides…and two cervix! Only since 2012 have I started receiving pap smears on each cervix, which should have been done since my first pap. I lost a little bit of faith in the medical community on that one.

Endometriosis is one of the leading causes of infertility. All of that time trying, crying, and fretting while we tried to make a baby…wasted. But at least now I know why I couldn't conceive.

But the BEST part? I have embraced this horrible disease and diagnosis, I've met beautiful and wonderfully passionate women who have the same disease, and we have come together for support and advocacy. I have learned that my pain was never normal. That I am not alone. And I have found a way to overcome the emotional shit-storm that came with the diagnosis.

I am stronger for it.

Words of Advice for Us: Having the love and support of your spouse, family, and friends is wonderful...but, I encourage you to find EndoSisters in your area, your community, your neck of the woods. Few things compare to being able relate with someone face-to-face, to hug, laugh out loud, see the pain in their eyes, be held as you try not to cry, share what has helped with your pain, relate to their pain, and have those "You, too???" moments. It is far better than any online support group and has made all of the difference in the world. Find a way to seek these women out. Go meet them! Don't wait for someone to start a group – start your own!

The Last Word: If you are feeling ugly, remember that you are still truly beautiful; inside and out. If you have no one to talk to, email or call me. You know your body like nobody else – if something doesn't feel right, tell your doctor. Insist. You're not crazy. And it's not normal.

If you wish to contact me, you can email me at lisa@bloominuterus.com or follow my blog.

Enough about me. I want to hear about you!

Yours, Lisa

Bloomin' Uterus is based out of San Diego, CA. I write for my blog, we started an Endometriosis support group in San Diego which now includes a lot of girls in Orange County and LA County and Riverside County and beyond...we have monthly support group meetings, host workshops with medical providers, and have an annual Endometriosis walk and fundraiser. I can't stop!

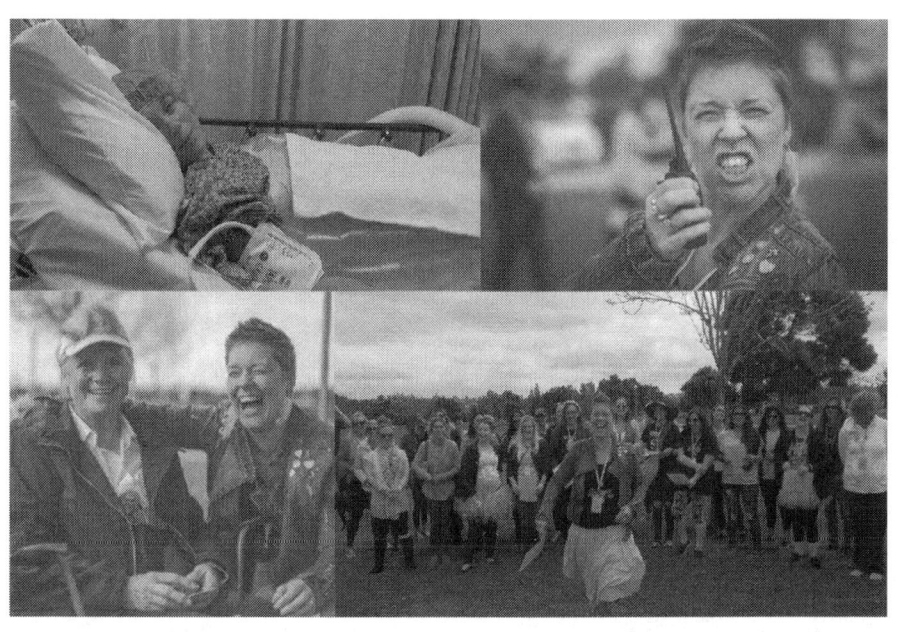

"The pain that you're in right now is not all in your head."

— Tricia Connelly

FIFTEEN

Tricia Connelly, Oklahoma

A Letter to My 12-Year-Old Self

My Dearest Tricia,

Well you are about to turn 37 years old.

I know life as a 12 year old is confusing right now. And that's okay.

Here's some things that you should know from me looking back.

I know when you look at women you have a funny feeling, like butterflies. That's ok, when you get old enough you will understand, you're a lesbian. Your best friend right now is Janett. And she gives you the butterflies. Tell her how you feel about her, and how she gives you the butterflies. She will tell you that she loves you too.

The pain that you're in right now is not all in your head, and it's not "just women pains" It's called endometriosis, not easy to say. Don't listen to the doctor. Get on some sort of pain medicine. Birth control pills are not going to work. Menstrual pain meds are not going to work either. Listen to our body. If something doesn't feel right to you DON'T DO IT!!!!!!!

On your 18th birthday DO NOT go to Bill's house. Not going to go into details. Just don't!!! Instead go out with your female friends. It'll be a lot more fun!

We are going to lose Carl to the Army. He's going to go to Iraq and fight in a war that America shouldn't be involved in. He will come home three times.

But on the fourth tour, he won't come home.

Keep him close and spend as much time with him that you can.

Much love,

Tricia

Facebook Support Groups
Admin, Gay Endo Sisters
Admin, Endometriosis Penpal Exchange
Admin, Endo Compilation Book 1 and 2

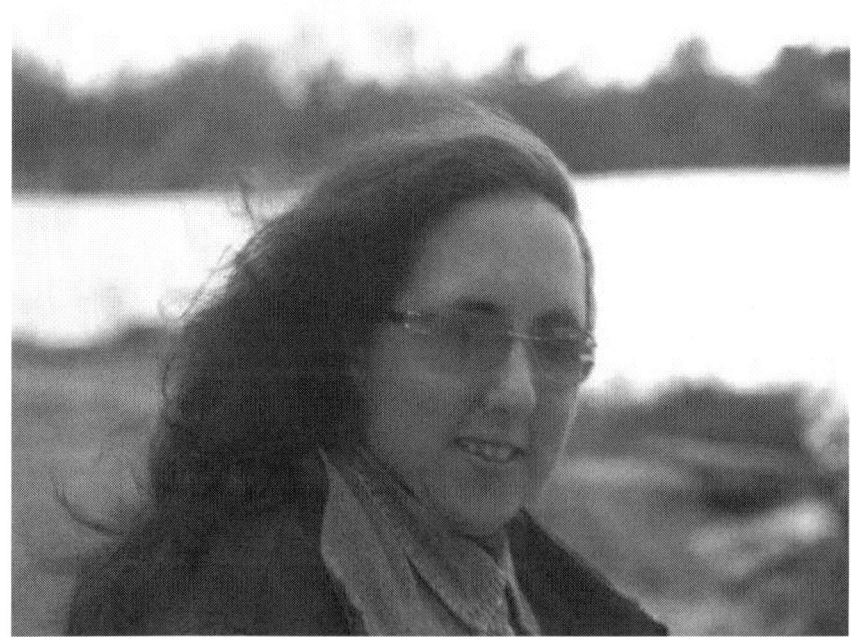

> "I was first symptomatic at age 15 with crippling pelvic and chest pain radiating to my legs, arms, temple, jaw and neck during my period. Then it started happening at ovulation too."
>
> – Cicely Daniels

SIXTEEN

Cicely Daniels, San Francisco Bay Area

My Endo Story

I was first symptomatic at age fifteen (1976) with crippling pelvic / chest pain radiating to my legs, arms, temple, jaw, neck, etc. during my period. Then it started happening at ovulation too.

By age nineteen I was going from doctor to doctor because my shoulder, neck, arms, and hands hurt all the time and some fingers had become numb. The tremendous arm, neck, shoulder pain was especially bad at night and when sitting down. Somehow I managed to finish classes at community college by recording (instead of using hands to write down) class notes, and standing in the back of the class instead of sitting. Unfortunately, after a successful transfer I subsequently had to drop out of Nursing school because the pain had became completely debilitating.

I also had to finally admit defeat and quit playing piano and guitar due to pain. I was very lost after that because my whole identity since a small child had revolved around being a musician and playing in bands.

Since the numerous doctors I saw could not figure out why I was so sick I started going to the biomedical library at UCLA (this was pre-Internet days) and I pulled journal articles looking for answers. Never once did I stumble across any articles about endometriosis and certainly not Thoracic endometriosis. I started doing alternative therapies as well looking for a way out of the pain. Acupuncture, meditation, Chinese medicine, diet. I tried anything anyone thought might help.

By now I had a slew of misdiagnosis under my belt. Asthma (only with period), Thoracic Outlet syndrome, Candida (very trendy back then), Porphyria (a chronic itchy rash and some weird lab values and anemia requiring transfusions prompted that one), mercury poisoning, various vitamin deficiencies, environmental sensitivity syndrome, migraine, crazy, hypochondriac ...

Then at age thirty a diagnostic laparoscopy was done and I was diagnosed with endometriosis in my Pelvic Cavity. Although my pelvic symptoms were severe, my Thoracic symptoms were the ones that completely dominated my life. No connection was made at that time and no pelvic endometriosis was excised just documented and burned superficially in a few spots.

To treat the pelvic endometriosis I started on birth control. Numerous different kinds were tried to control the bleeding and pain. The side effects were nausea and headache all the time and they did not work to control my endo pain. Then Depot Provera was tried. Those three sequential shots caused me to bleed non-stop for two years straight. Nothing stopped the bleeding from that drug until at a coworker's suggestion, I saw a Chinese professor (college of acupuncture Santa Monica) who gave me herbs to drink four times daily for a week.

Some more time passed, a second Pelvic surgery by a more skilled OBGYN doctor who only did ablation. Disease in bladder and chest were not looked for and thus missed completely.

Still very sick, Depot Lupron therapy was initiated. Two weeks into the first shot both sides of my chest started burning uncontrollably and I could not breathe. I was told it was a severe asthma attack and I actually quit my job thinking it was a reaction to the chemicals in the job environment. I stayed on Lupron the next six years as it did control my pelvic symptoms. It did not control the Thoracic issues but they were diagnosed as Thoracic outlet so no one expected them too.

I moved to the Bay Area and had another pelvic surgery with a even more skilled surgeon, Dr. Nezhat at Stanford. He was able to remove endometriosis from typical pelvic locations inside bladder wall, ureters, Pouch of Douglas, etc.

About a year after that surgery, I started coughing blood with my period. When I mentioned this to Dr. Nezhat he immediately suspected Thoracic endometriosis. This was pre-VATs time so he proposed a open chest procedure to excise the endometriosis. To avoid that horrible procedure I tried a gluten-free endometriosis diet. My rash I'd had since a baby went away, so did the stomach aches I thought were from endometriosis. Anemia and the other slew of weird vitamin deficiencies resolved. I was finally able to gain to a normal body weight. So all those things were very positive but the crippling acute monthly 36 hours straight uncontrollable pain, vomiting, and suffocation of Thoracic endo flares continued.

Still trying to avoid chest surgery the "new" aromatase inhibitor drugs were tried. Within three days the chest pain eased dramatically, but within a week the crippling arthralgia side effects started. After six weeks I was unable to continue the medication as I could not sleep nor walk due to the severe arthralgia side effects.

I went back to Stanford (2010) and was the 19th patient to have a team of doctors there do a combination LAP/ Bilateral VATS (newly available) surgery. Thirty eight endometriosis nodules were treated with Fulguration (another term for ablation) from the Pulmonary side of my diaphragm. Majority right sided (32), remainder (6) from the left side.

After recovery from this surgery. I felt so tremendously good. The first time in decades. Unfortunately, due to the fact that the Thoracic disease was ablated instead of excised I had disease recurrence within the year. I also learned I had suspected Adenomyosis (endometriosis in the uterine wall). The only treatment available for that was hysterectomy or menopause. Being 45 years old at the time I opted to avoid additional surgery and wait until menopause, which was assumed would cause resolution of Adenomyosis symptoms.

After that recurrence, my Thoracic phrenic nerve pathway pain/ Respiratory distress pattern of continued severe 24/7 and the cyclical acute 36-hour uncontrollable pain exacerbations persisted monthly despite access to high-dose narcotic therapy. By that time, five-years post-menopausal and another trial of progesterone/aromatase inhibitor therapy for 18 months. High vitamin D therapy with the aromatase inhibitors controlled the arthralgia symptoms a good 65%.

So at this point between the narcotics and the aromatase inhibitors and the strategy of resting all the time when not at work I was able to keep my job and by extension my health insurance. No quality of life though and the cyclic exacerbations prompted repeated incidences paramedics being called and ER visits for oxygen/ IV pain control and feelings of suffocation/ out-of-breath, all the time.

Enter Facebook and Nancy's Nook Endometriosis Education Group. I learned about the marked difference in recurrence rates between Excision surgery and Fulguration/ Ablation surgery. I also got access to the international list of excision endometriosis specialist doctors. These types of doctors have extensive extra surgical training and experience compared to the OBGYNs most women see. Excision specialist doctors treat endometriosis patients as focus of their practice and work as a team with other specialists to excise extra pelvic disease.

I was referred from a member of that site to another support group for women with Thoracic endometriosis. It was life changing because members on that site told me about the Center for Endometriosis care in Atlanta Georgia. CEC offered an experienced multidisciplinary team approach to treating endometriosis. Very importantly they had experience routinely treating endometriosis in the Pulmonary system by excising it completely.

No one anywhere on the West Coast did this procedure, so in September 2017 I flew to Atlanta for a combination right sided VATs / LAP procedure to excise the right sided diaphragm endometriosis recurrence. I also had a partial hysterectomy to finally treat my adenomyosis which had continued cycling pain unabated despite being at that point five years post menopause.

I woke up from that operation being able to breathe for the first time in years. So far I have not had any cyclical endo flares on the right side. Treating the adenomyosis eliminated my remaining pelvic pain / constant urinary urgency. Both are now a thing of the past.

After forty-one years of trying everything anyone suggested to stop the cyclical pain from this disease, the only area of my body that continues to cycle is the left side of my chest where some endo remains untreated. That pain is monthly but so far controllable as well as it appears all my respiratory distress was coming from the right sided diaphragm endometriosis. A left sided VATs will be needed to treat the remaining left sided disease as bilateral VATs excision is not done at this point. Treating bilateral diaphragm disease takes two separate VATs procedures.

When I feel physically / mentally ready to undergo another chest surgery I will fly back to Atlanta to get the left sided disease excised. So far no respiratory distress from that side. The left sided pain is not 24/7 only cyclical, so compared to what the right side of my chest put me through I am taking it a day at a time as far as committing to the next surgery. I continue to get stronger with each passing day and am enjoying immensely my new free of continuous pain and being able to breathe life.

I am no longer trapped isolated in pain, suffocating. I am also learning to actually make plans with friends to do things and go places besides work and doctors offices. Making plans and fun are things I had stopped doing years ago as previous to VATs excision of the diaphragm endo, any increased activity and talking exacerbated my pain severely.

I have started singing again without pain too which is a miracle for me. Oh and I can lay down now without suffocating. For years I slept sitting up. My wedge pillow has been officially retired!

I am happy to share my story if it will help spread awareness about endometriosis and how important getting treatment from a specialist team that does complete with clean margins excision. This is currently the most (in my humble opinion, the only) effective treatment available for this disease. Particularly extra-pelvic locations like the respiratory system.

If my story helps others avoid what I went through then there is some meaning / purpose to my decades long battle of constant pain / respiratory distress from Thoracic / Pelvic locations Endometriosis / Adenomyosis.

> "The status of endo care worldwide is criminal. Every woman deserves relief from this kind of pain."
>
> – Nancy Petersen, RN

SEVENTEEN

Nancy Petersen (RN), Oregon

Living with Life-Altering Pain - October 2012

A little background on why I think I can write this article: from the time I was 10 or 11 years old, I have pretty much been in pain. Daily.

By the time I was 27, I still did not have a diagnosis and was in so much pain, all I could do was work and try to get enough rest so I could work again the next day. My low back and left leg were in continuous pain, to the extent that I could sleep only about 4-6 hrs a night.

Then I had my 3rd episode of acute abdominal pain and was hospitalized, and a gyn consultant called. To his credit, he diagnosed endo after doing a pelvic exam, and as usual, during the exam, I was willing to leave the table with the speculum still in place. He did not mimic my internal medicine specialist, saying: "calm down, pelvic exams do not hurt!", but instead said, "I always watch my patient's face when I do a pelvic exam. This tells me everything." Dr. Redwine mentioned this too about watching patients faces while doing the exam.

"Enovid," he said (an older birth control pill), "triple dose. If this doesn't do it, come by the office and we will talk about a hysterectomy."

I discussed it with the OB/GYN head nurse, who suggested another opinion if it came to that. This was in the days before GnRH agonists. Finally, my pain was so severe, and blood loss so great, I got my second opinion and opted for a complete hysterectomy.

Because of the back and leg pain, now having reduced my sleeping to two hours a night, I also saw an orthopedist who said: "since your hysterectomy didn't help your back pain, you need a laminectomy and fusion of your low back". Mind you, this was 1969, and I was sort of meek in those days. So - I had one of those, too.

For the next 22 years, my back and leg pain bore a hole in my mind, my soul, my life. Sleep came in 20-minute parcels. It seemed to me this was my lot. Gradually, I began having significant bowel and bladder pain, and about 16 years into this period of pain, I began lecturing on endometriosis and Modern Concepts as developed by Dr. Redwine (Bend, Oregon). As I traveled around North America lecturing, I would stay as long as the questions flowed about endo and Modern Concepts. Often, I would hear stories of pain that were so similar I began to wonder if I still had endo. Mind you, it was not a common understanding that endo could persist or recur following a complete hysterectomy then.

"Gee, that sounds like me", I would say to myself.

During those 22 years after the hyst, I had only myself to rely on. I had to work, often long hours as I was first a critical care nurse, then a house supervisor and upper manager, and then spent 22 weeks a year on the road visiting support groups teaching Modern Concepts. I was on my feet, all the while, with pain so severe it broke through my every action, thought, attempt to sleep; it stole my relationship, in many ways the joy in my life. I had to find a way to least find something in life that was positive.

I began a series of self-care attempts. I spent a great deal of money on massage, acupuncture, acupressure, Rolfing, Feldenkrais, chiropractic, and naturopathic care. The book, "Free Yourself from Pain" by David Bresler, Ph.D. became my bible. I literally tried most of the stuff in that book, including visualization, relaxation training, hypnosis, drawing and writing my pain, counseling, group supports. My mantra was if it is not likely to hurt me, not outrageously expensive, and not just plain stupid, I would try it.

Some things I learned: first, current pain is almost always linked to other primal pains such as parental abandonment, abuse (physical, mental, emotional, etc.), low self esteem, isolation, loneliness, and a host of other issues – or maybe, just bad medical care and refusal to believe us! So if you were victimized by other events or abuses in your life, you may well feel victimized by endometriosis; another learning point was while pain may be a major factor in your life, there are many ways to distract your mind, finding ways to nurture yourself can help alter the brain's focus. My reading helped my learning; however, I also chose to spend time with a counselor to aid my learning.

The key issue here is the 'state of the art' is, in fact, such a sorry state. When we do not experience improvement with ineffective treatment we must be nuts, right? Of course it is easier for caregivers to believe we are neurotic than to accept there is something wrong with basic endo care. 75% of the patients we saw had been dismissed as neurotic, after multiple medical and surgical treatment failures. ALL had biopsy proven disease as determined by board certified independent pathologists from the tissue Dr. Redwine and Dr. Sharp submitted.

A recent series of articles in a special edition of health news by the Bend Bulletin revealed that over half of the research appearing worldwide in medical journals, news releases, medical conferences, even coming out of universities is WRONG. This is a critical observation and is even worse in women with endo. So we are challenged to survive until quality care is available to all of us, and the maltreatment offered as the standard fare has been banned from medicine forever.

I began to carry a small cassette recorder/player (who knew the age of iPods was just around the corner) around with me, and when I took my breaks, I would spend 20 minutes in deep relaxation, and then be able to go on for a while longer. Computer solitaire was invented for my sleepless nights. Music with a headset so as not to disturb others in the house was also helpful, as was late night chats online, research online, anything that put my mind somewhere other than the blistering pain in my belly and mind-boring pain in my calf.

I became a prolific reader of self care, alternative care, ways of distracting the mind. Guess what? All that reading, video watching, tape listening, helped move my brain out of the continuous focus on the pain.

On of the books I read was "Flow, the Psychology of Optimal Experience" by Mihaly Csikszentmihalyi. While it was written in a very scholastic way, I was able to pick out some key ideas, one of which is when you get into something you truly love, your life flows and distractions can be minimized in the moment. I began gardening. Raised-bed gardening was something I had been reading about, as well as reading a book by Ruth Stout, "The No Work Garden Book." I found ways to adapt my life and my garden so I could still do this without making my life and pain worse.

This gave me back some power over my life.

During this time, no one was helping me with pain; we did not even know what was wrong with me, especially since the fusion did not help. So as my joy at digging my hands into the soil, particularly in an extremely difficult climate, began to emerge, I found that I could forget the pain for minutes, sometimes, half hours at a time. Even today, although my endo pain has been resolved, genetic malformations in my spine have taken center court, but I can put the pain aside for hours at a time, by finding joy. This is NOT to say the pain goes away, but rather the brain is trained to look elsewhere for periods of time.

I do not believe I would have had the strength to persist if my endometriosis had not been resolved through excision, given the progressive, genetic defect in my upper back. So I am grateful for the success of endo removal. I did eventually undergo expert excision of endo found on the uterosacral ligaments, pelvic floor, and pelvic sidewalls, 22 years post "curative hysterectomy" it took 2.5 hrs to remove the rest of my endo.

You cannot just muscle through the pain. Sometimes that will make things worse because you work physically beyond your tolerance, but you can distract the mind from paying attention for periods of time. Is it easy? Not at all! It is hard work, requiring self-education, focus, practice - and sometimes you will fail. In some cases, you may always fail! BUT trying to improve your ability to cope with pain until you can find more effective care can be empowering, and give you a sense of purpose.

Please do not interpret this to mean you can always do 'mind over matter' where your pain is concerned. Rather, you can build in short respites, sometimes even longer. For me, it was at least something I could try. That alone was empowering.

Hear me: your pain is as REAL and severe as acute appendicitis can be (I know, I had both) - only it is chronic, continuous, mind-boring, and you always deserve better care than is offered to the 176,000,000 women worldwide.

The status of endo care worldwide is criminal. Every woman deserves relief from this kind of pain. It takes more skill than most surgeons have, but it is not beyond their ability to learn if they seek skilled mentors.

So what is holding them back?

Nancy Petersen-RN, Retired

Facebook/Nancy's Nook Endometriosis Education
60,000 members
Volunteer, Endometriosis Research Center

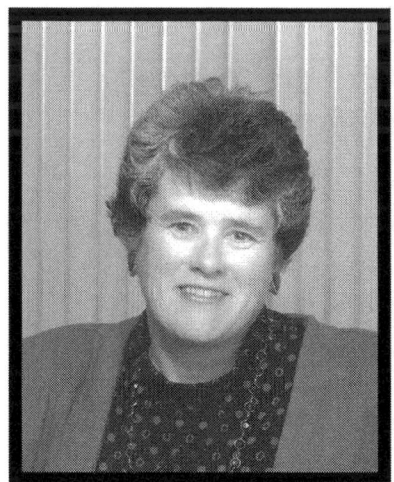
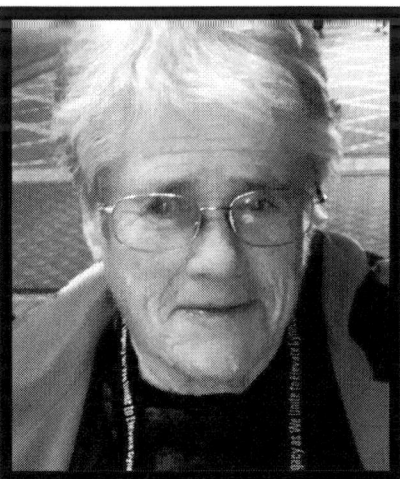

> "Every month thousands of patients report not being believed, disease left behind, being told it was not there or that it was inoperable, or that it would cause permanent damage to try to remove it, or that it would dry up and go away if we just take out your ovaries, or your uterus or both, is just unacceptable. Can't be that bad you say? Indeed it is worse than that."
>
> – *Nancy Petersen, RN*

Endometriosis: Lead, Follow, or Get Out of the Way, daily failed treatments

An open letter by Nancy Petersen.

I do not know what else to say. That gynecology in large numbers leaves symptomatic endometriosis while offering ineffective care is stunning. It matters not whether endometriosis is stage 1 or deeply invasive disease, if it hurts, almost nothing gynecology has to offer will alleviate the suffering short of removing the causative factors.

But to mislead patients as to the presence of disease, occurring regularly among our patient population is a stunning finding. Every month thousands of patients report not being believed, disease left behind, being told it was not there or that it was inoperable, or that it would cause permanent damage to try to remove it, or that it would dry up and go away if we just take out your ovaries, or your uterus or both, is just unacceptable.

Can't be that bad you say? Indeed it is worse than that.

Treatment of endometriosis is an abusive black eye in medicine for the most part with the exception of those teaching MIGS, and endo-specific skills in patient care. Senator Hatch from Utah calls it a national epidemic, while accurate, it is a silent epidemic allowing gynecology to continue blithely on ignoring their own shortcomings, protecting their members incomes while overlooking the disease's impact.

The denial of the devastation these patients face is pathological, abusive and may border on malpractice. I do not suggest this lightly, the only thing that permits gynecology to continue on this course of ineffective medical, surgical, (including ablation, hysterectomy, castration, central sensitization referrals, psychological dismissal) therapies is to ignore the reality of the impact of this disease on patients lives as well as their family, friends, and colleagues. Peritoneal quality pain is severe, disabling, destroying sexuality, careers, daily life relationships, fertility, and any other aspect of life.

The repeated shifting the focus to psychological states while leaving painful peritoneal and or organ disease in place is a pass for surgeons who cannot manage this disease effectively. Without exception patients struggle emotionally when peritoneal quality pain is present that impact quality of sleep, sex, normal bodily functions like bowel movements or full bladder, the ability to exercise, to procreate, to have a career, to maintain relationships, but it is not the primary illness. The primary illness is pain, severe pain that no medical student or nursing student on the planet should overlook but regularly do. Peritoneal signs and symptoms are commonly recognized and respected except in women with endometriosis, endometriomas, PCOS, adenomyosis, where somehow we shift to: "Oh, it's just her period."

Suppressive drugs subject patients to low estrogen states, putting them at risk for small vessel heart disease, stroke, bone loss, memory impairment, and generally a lack of well being. Lost on gynecology is that patients do not like altered hormonal states. Do the physicians not care? There are options you know, to remove disease with proper training that reduces risks and relieves symptoms as well as reducing or eliminating the need for altered hormonal states via suppressive drugs. Yet ACOG resists recognizing the lack of adequate management.

They have yet to endorse the need to stop removal of normal ovaries and uteruses, and they continue to overlook the impact of laparotomies and their potential for complications, delayed recovery.

They also are apparently in denial that removal of normal organs and leaving endometriosis elsewhere is not an effective strategy in endometriosis management. We continue to shake our heads in amazement that a group of science-based physicians can believe that removing normal organs while leaving disease elsewhere could have some positive impact on the health of these patients.

When ACOG does gather to discuss, they conveniently leave recognized experts out of the conversation. What is the motivation for failing to include those who are getting long-lasting to permanent relief of symptoms? Does big pharma free flowing dollars impact science? I suggest it closes science out of the conversation entirely. Big pharma paying for articles, and then doing the editing of them raises serious concerns about who is looking after the patients.

We recognize that hormonal therapies have a role in certain conditions, but it is very clear there is no evidence that any medication treats endometriosis and now we are on the verge of a whole new bevy of ineffective drugs offering unacceptable hormonal states and side effect are about to be sprung on endometriosis patients world wide.

Everyone is sooo excited, except the patients. They know full well it is another dead end, where physicians will push drugs that do not work and from at least some big pharma who have a history of hiding actual side effects so that physicians and patients alike cannot possible have full understanding of the ramifications of taking GnRH medications.

Then when serious side effect crop up, physicians continue to be very critical of the patients reports, telling them there is no evidence that this could be true. (Because evidence was suppressed by court order)

In groups like ours where we have some 40,000 patients who have failed all gynecology has to offer, there is little doubt about the seriousness of the side effects with thousands of reports of side effects now lingering years after the medication was stopped. As well, original study data analysis showed that the company under reported both the number and seriousness of the side effects (this is the report big pharma hid with a court order and the FDA bowed down). Over 10,000 reports have been submitted to the FDA on side effects. Still patients experiences are denied by their caregivers.

While other pelvic pain generators do exist, they too can be identified and treatment plans developed. The lack of motivation to properly care for patients is stunning among a group that should be science based as well as compassionate in patient care.

Again, we implore ACOG to lead, follow or get out of the way, at least if nothing else join AAGL in pushing for training for less invasive surgeries, more effective removal of disease and stop doing harm. It's time you are held accountable.

"Endometriosis is Latin for: doctor thinks I'm crazy; gynecologist can't find it, and family thinks I am a loser."

– Brandi LaPerle

EIGHTEEN

Brandi CK LaPerle, Canada

Open Letter to Doctors

Dear Doctors,

Endometriosis is known to be one of the most painful human experiences known to medicine unrelated to child-bearing or cancer.

Endometriosis affects more patients than asthma, diabetes, and breast cancer combined. There is no recognition or compassion for the crippling invisible disease which leaves patients feeling lost, confused, invalidated, and in a state of despair.

They look fine on the outside, but their insides are literally at war! A smile may be there, but the blisters and lesions inside create acute inflammation which develops scar tissue and adhesions that infiltrate organs and can even bind them together. Scar tissue and musculoskeletal distortion to compensate for organs being glued together pulling in different directions for years without treatment can cause ongoing acute pain even after lesions are removed.

The resulting symptoms can involve pain during bowel movements, pain during sex (sexual arousal alone can be painful), damage to the nervous system, pain during bladder void, nausea, vomiting, migraine, and so much more!

Endometriosis is rarely found alone. Numerous co-morbid conditions include: fibromyalgia, PCOS, fibroids, lupus, pelvic floor dysfunction, adenomyosis, chronic fatigue, endocrine dysfunction, atopic disease, interstitial cystitis, autoimmune disease, pudendal neuralgia, gastrointestinal disease, and so much more!

The disease affects the reproductive system, so women are often treated medically with barbarism. We know hysterectomy isn't an effective treatment, yet I meet so many young vibrant women with so much life ahead that have been butchered by multiple failed ablations (cauterization of the surface of the disease with 80% fail rate) and have had their organs removed only to learn later when the pain/symptoms continue to worsen that it was medically unnecessary.

I've met patients with organs removed as young as 16–18 suffering because they trusted their gynecologist knew the best way to alleviate their pain.

Sadly, we have learned gynecologists have a narrow lesson on treating complex incurable disease like endometriosis in their training based on archaic methods known to have high failure rates. Patients need to know there are options available to them and empowered to make the best decision for their care. Each patient's journey and case is different and no one treatment is good for every patient in the world.

Care absolutely requires individualized multidisciplinary and psychosocial approach to management since there is no cure. Medical professionals from various disciplines involved in a patient's care need to communicate amongst one another effectively and involve the patient in the decision-making process.

Each doctor involved needs to know the patient experience is real. Hormonal therapies that can only serve as a temporary band-aid and other medications can be highly expensive with side effects for many worse than the disease itself. When these therapies fail the patient is often blamed for this failure! What are they doing wrong in their life? This is unacceptable.

At least you don't have cancer though. Oh how those words cut like a knife through the soul of a woman fighting for an inch of hope.

Suffering is no competition! There is no gold medal for having it worse, or knowing someone that does.

Cancer patients with endometriosis are not staying silent on this! Many have stepped forward to share their brave story of fighting cancer with the pressure to become an inspirational story to be shared on facebook to make those around them feel better. These patients insist their pain from endometriosis is often worse than their breast cancer, ovarian cancer, and various other recognizable devastating illnesses we identify. They share their story of how their pain was never validated until they had cancer because the world knows how devastating it is even though they had suffered for years prior only to be silenced.

Let us not make comparisons for suffering! Let us just recognize that endometriosis alone impacts every facet of a patient's life mentally, emotionally, sexually, spiritual, and absolutely physically.

Don't silence her voice.

When patients share their stories in social media to raise awareness to help others to understand, they are bombarded by angry messages demanding they drop the negativity and seek mental health care. You wouldn't do that to a person with asthma, diabetes, or cancer. For some reason it is perfectly acceptable when the disease affects the reproductive organs of a female.

In rare cases the disease also affects some men that don't have a uterus (fancy that!). We have men in Canada ashamed to raise their voices because Endometriosis is still, in many respects, seen as the hysterical woman's womb disease.

Endometriosis can be found anywhere in the body. In our local, national, and global support groups we have patients with endometriosis pathologically diagnosed on the lungs, diaphragm, and even the heart.

Yet, these patients spent the same average 11 years going from doctor to doctor being told there was nothing wrong with them! It was ALL in their head. Just a painful period! Prescribed antidepressants and given referral to psychiatrist for evaluation. Gynecologists performed laparoscopic surgery only identifying a small fraction of the various presentations of endometriosis and scarring throughout their bodies. Most only look closely at the reproductive organs telling the patient there is no cause for their continued pain.

Endometriosis is Latin for: doctor thinks I'm crazy, gynecologist can't find it, and family thinks I'm a loser.

Alternative definition: Angry gorilla on bath salts attacking the inside of the body.

Family, friends, and significant others struggle to understand the struggle many patients endure. Some experience no pain only to gain diagnosis during another procedure or when fertility becomes a concern (endometriosis is a top cause of infertility).

This means that those suffering great pain with severe symptoms can be marginalized by others with the disease that fail to understand how it can vary from patient to patient. Some will have had a hysterectomy for mild endometriosis and insist a patient whose options are very limited should just get one to cure them.

This misinformed dismissive approach only serves to further isolate the patient that needs nothing more than extra love and compassion as they muster every bit of courage to keep on fighting for the care they need.

Many patients must travel thousands of miles to gain the skilled hand required to address the complexity of their case. The costs astronomical and the risks of traveling post-surgery are real. For these patients the cost is an investment for hope of a quality of life in their future.

Excision surgery is recognized by the global leaders in endometriosis care and research as being the gold standard of treatment. Very few gynecologists around the world have undertaken the difficult training to achieve successful long-term outcomes for patients. MOST of the gynecologists I've talked to in the last three years are NOT familiar with this procedure. They do NOT even know of the rare few with the skill to perform it!

Endometriosis is often described as a benign cancer-like disease that, in rare cases, knows how to metastasize itself. I've met one patient in Alberta with this rare occurrence and nobody in the medical field would believe her story. It was proven through biopsy, medical testing, and pathology, but she remained stigmatized by those she depended on to help her because their knowledge was too limited despite the evidence before them. She had absolutely no compassion for care until it was cancer.

Even when it is not cancer, the disease can sometimes be progressive. Organs can be infiltrated and damaged, but there is no urgency for care.

Being partnered with Worldwide EndoMarch I learned that severe chronic pain (as what endometriosis patients frequently experience) is responsible for up to 70% of suicides. I've shown this statistic to medical professionals that refute the claims although they agree the researchers are reliable.

"That's a joke. Endometriosis is not my job. I'm an ER doctor and there is not one good reason a patient with this disease should ever have to be seen in the ER." – Edmonton, Alberta ER physician

The week I spoke to this doctor I had lost 9 women to either complications or giving up due to medical dismissal of the severity of their symptoms. They reached out for help. They sought emergency mental health support.

I get the call at 1am from a tearful parent that says "she lost her battle." These patients that would normally be stigmatized gain recognition which scares me, dear Doctors. They never get to hear those words of validation that they were ever fighting a battle at all.

I must keep this information very private and rarely speak of it to my community because I don't want others to follow. I must mourn quietly because I know how much she suffered, but cannot let others feel this is an option.

There is HOPE! It doesn't have to be this way. She doesn't have to suffer like that. No parent should have to learn the depth of her despair and suffering by losing a child when its too late to hold him/her.

In the US the estimate cost to taxpayers is $119 BILLION. In Canada the estimated cost to taxpayers (that's you) is $1.5 BILLION.

These costs are accrued due to the systemic failure in effectively treating disease and years of delay for diagnosis.

The pain can be worse than childbirth at any time, or all of the time (as was my own experience). The exhaustion similar to that of some end stage cancers.

The cause is UNKNOWN (this means there are theories, but there is no known cause if anyone tries to claim they know)
There is NO cure! (beware of those that seek to exploit the vulnerability of desperate patients)

Hysterectomy will NOT treat endometriosis!

What can YOU do to help?

If you or someone you know has Endometriosis please let them know about Alberta Endo Group on Facebook. Let them know about Endoisreal.org. Let them know about Worldwide EndoMarch.
Listen. Do not compare!

Do not tell her to be positive.

Be compassionate.

Recognize that she is TRULY suffering due to NO fault of her own.

Step away from the doctor shows and google claims of having a treatment or cure.

Offer to help.

You are not alone in this battle and ENDO IS REAL!

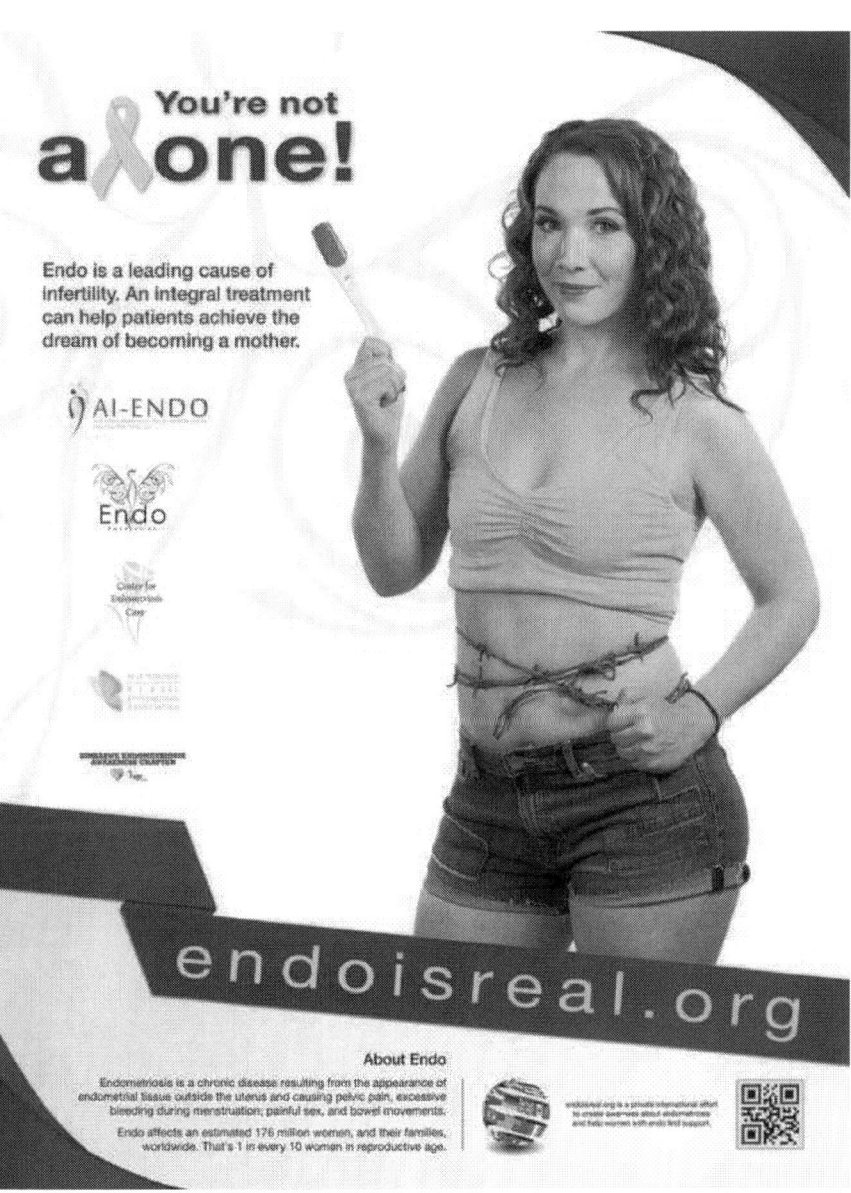

> "I was written up (at work). They said I needed to get this under control or I may lose my job due to my attendance. But I couldn't help the stabbing pain."
>
> – Stephany Adeyemi

NINETEEN

Stephany Adeyemi, Texas

I was thirteen the first time I had a "bad cramp". From then on they never went away and just got worse. I would double over in pain. Movement in general while having a cramp just made it worse like a nerve being shocked in my abdominal area. I would just have to stay still until the cramp passed.

I would ask to stay home from school during the first day or two, and luckily a few times my grandmother let me. I tried things like Midol and other off-the-shelf pain meds, but they didnt do a damn thing. It was like I just ate a piece of candy to try to manage my cramps, no relief.

When I was fourteen years old we went to a doctor and talked about my cramps and I was prescribed Ponstel. It's a prescription pain medication specifically for menstrual cramps. It worked and I just stayed on it for a few years. But over the years my cramps were getting worse, and the medication wasn't always helping. I started taking a double dose of it on the bad days just because it was the only thing that helped. That was against my doctor's instructions, but I had to ease the pain. I had to start adding some Advil in the evenings until again, nothing helped.

I missed work at times and asked to go home, because I just couldn't walk without that shooting, stabbing pain with every movement. My managers gave me a hard time about it because they didn't think it was "that bad" and I got written up for these occurrences. It came to a point that they sat down with me in the office and talked about how I needed to get this under control or I may lose my job due to my attendance. But I couldn't help that I needed to be off a few days out of the month. I wished they could understand it was real.

I went to the doctor and just got more of the same, birth control, extra strength Ibuprofen, "Don't know what's wrong with you."

From age nineteen to twenty five, my fiance and I (at the time) attempted to have children. It never happened. I tried all of the things you hear "help" short of fertility treatments, which I didn't have the money for. He would say things like how he didn't want to be with someone who couldn't have his kids. Granted he was a jerk and it ultimately didn't work out, but it stuck with me. I felt defective, broken.

When I started dating my now husband I told him right off the bat about my issues and that I couldn't have kids. I'd accepted that as a fact at this point.

At age thirty-one I went to the doctor about pain in my ovary area (again). I wasn't able to have intercourse without severe pain. This was taking an emotional toll on me, because I felt inadequate when it came to my husband. Now to clarify he has been nothing but wonderful, understanding & supportive. This was just my own feeling about the situation.

The doctor checked me out in every way possible – did ultrasounds, exams, gave me medication, all that he could think of, but nothing changed. He did find that my left ovary was three times the size it should have been, because it wasn't working properly, which explained the ovary pain. He put me on birth control to help regulate that issue and it worked for a year. Except that I kept ending up with multiple infections and the painful intercourse never went away, it got worse.

I asked to be referred to another doctor, because this one just scratched his head saying he couldn't figure me out and just simply didn't think I had endometriosis. He told me that maybe because I was expecting to feel the pain that my mind was telling me that I felt the pain. He was actually suggesting that it was in my head. He wouldn't even talk about going in to see for sure. His words were "surgery is a pretty radical idea."

Finally receiving a referral was the best thing ever. This new doctor asked me a bunch of questions I'd never been asked in relation to my pain. Did I have migraines? For how long? When did the cramps start? Did I always have a heavy period? He asked about my ovary issues, the painful intercourse. He did an examination, which was always very painful, and this concerned him more than I had seen any other doctor be concerned.

During that first visit this doctor told me he believed I had endometriosis and was scheduling me for a laparoscopic surgery. Laparoscopy is the ONLY WAY to 100% confirm a woman has endometriosis. It does not show up on x-rays or ultrasounds. To say that being told I was being scheduled for surgery made my day is pretty sad, but it meant answers and I'd been searching for half of my life.

When I woke up from surgery the first words out of my mouth were "did you find anything?" Because I had to know that there was some reason for feeling this way. I had to know there was something wrong and it wasn't in my head.

What this doctor found was, in his words, "one of the most severe cases of stage 4 endometriosis" he'd ever seen. My abdominal organs were so covered in endometriosis tissue that they were knitted together and had to be separated. My right ovary had been destroyed, and he couldn't separate my uterus from my rectal area due to possible damage to those muscles which would result in me needing to use a colostomy bag.

But I was relieved, I had an answer. I knew what was wrong with me. I was going to need another surgery though.

But first I had to take a six-month treatment that put me into a medical menopause to help "dry up" the endometriosis. Estrogen feeds endometriosis and makes it grow, so he needed to stop the growth before he could attempt another surgery. He told me that so much damage had been done that I had been rendered infertile and he recommended a hysterectomy.

My right ovary was dead tissue and the right tube also crushed and non functioning. My left ovary and tube were almost to that same point. And the severity to which my uterus was fused to my rectum would have made it impossible to carry a child were I to miraculously conceive. The weight of anything in my uterus would have most likely caused it to tear away from the fusion and cause severe damage along with miscarriage.

A part if me always knew though, that I would never be able to become pregnant, so this wasn't a shocker. He said that after seeing my insides that he believed I had had this since I was about thirteen. Those first cramps I had were the first signs I had endometriosis. And if anyone of those doctors I had seen and begged for help over those seventeen years would have taken action and believed, me my insides could have been saved.

It took five doctors, from age thirteen to age thirty-one to figure out what was wrong with me. And by then the damage had already been done. I went through the very expensive treatment of being in medical menopause for six months and had a hysterectomy. It took two surgeons to be able to save my bowels, and for me not end up with the colostomy bag. What was expected to be a two-hour surgery at max was over four hours.

Recovery went well and for the first time in my life I'm pain free. In fact I was so grateful for being able to feel "normal" that I actually cried tears of joy and relief when it set in.

My biggest fear though is the pain returning, having to prove to all over again, because there is no cure for endometriosis.

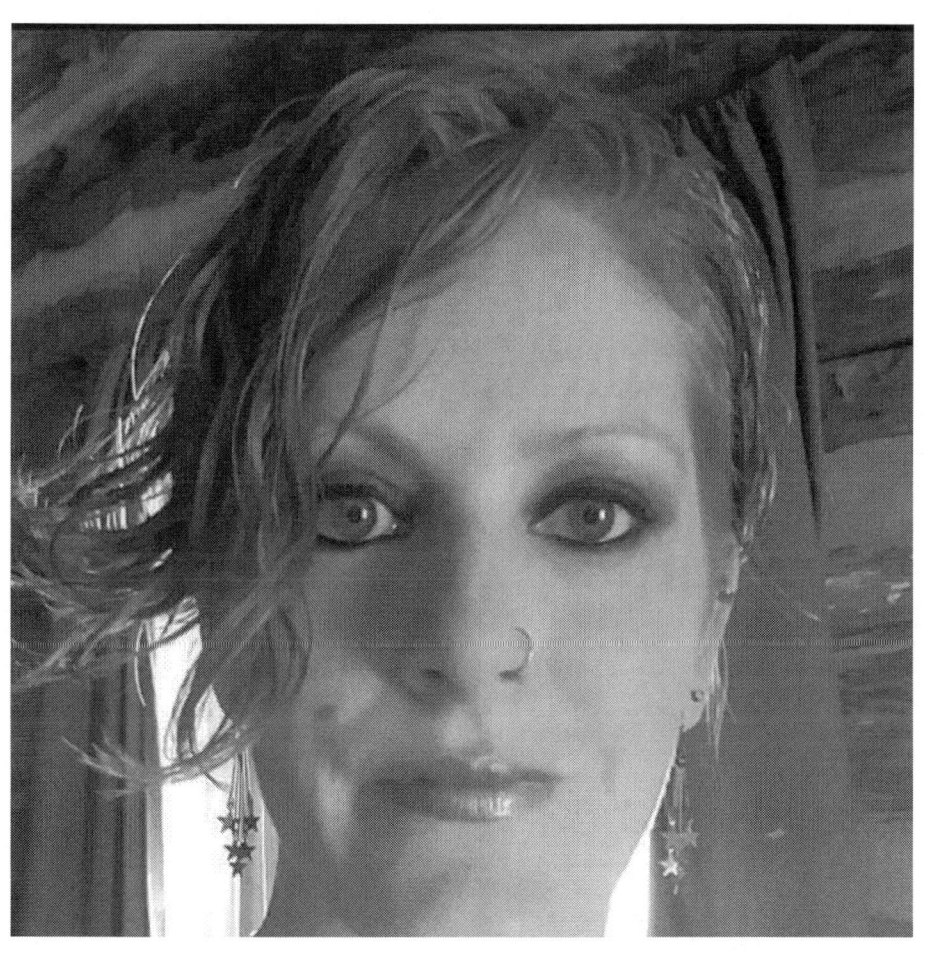

"Endometriosis is a thief. It steals days and months. It steals years of our lives."

– Jaimee Rae McCormack

TWENTY and TWENTY ONE

Jaimee Rae McCormack & Laura Mccormack-Long
Cardiff, United Kingdom

EndoWall, The Rising Awareness

"You realise the pain is just in your head don't you? It's psychosomatic so try not to worry about it."

Thirteen years searching for a diagnosis and the GPs still don't believe me… I know the brain is a powerful tool but this pain is not in my head!

I decline his suggestion of antidepressants and take my frustration home, submerging back into Google…

10th March - Endometriosis awareness Day - why didn't I know that?

I call upon a friend with a camera and I dress in yellow from my headphones to my shoes. The side of my house forms the wall of a lane. At first a crying yellow ribbon appears and then I spray 'ENDOMETRIOSIS EXISTS' a metre high with a can of black spray paint. Robin French clicks and snaps from every angle. Giant yellow sunflowers escape from the can like a genie. Nine golden petals evolve, then a solitary black one to represent the one in ten women cursed to live with the chronic pain of Endometriosis…every month of our lives -from puberty to menopause.

My energy reservoir and cans are empty, I slump to the ground. 'So fuckin' disrespectful! I don't wanna look at that shit everyday!' A guy ten years younger is screaming at me.

Fighting back tears I try to explain.

He has zero interest.

My spirit breaks.

Robin continues to click and snap.

These images are the most powerful.

The lad spits on the floor, turns and leaves.

Waking feeling older than it says on paper, I rest as my body tells me to. The hours tick by, but before I know it I'm buying more spray paints and returning to my mission.

The cans glint and shoosh in the glare of the lamppost as my wrist twists and my finger guides.

Yellow, black, black, more and more yellow.

Suddenly rays of flashing blue lights are bouncing off the walls.
I panic. Walk the other way.

'Miss!'

I increase my pace.

'We've had a report of vandalism to this property!'

I can't outrun them, my limbs heavy like oak trunks.

'Oh no that's ok. It's my house.'

'Really? That's a first! Would you be kind enough to prove that for us please Miss?'

My key unlocks the door and I enjoy the shift.

Unlike the lad in the lane they show interest...(well they were in my house so their ears couldn't get away!) One officer already knows Endo, they're helpful and kind and laugh when I explain …

'To be arrested would really bring publicity. I need it. This could really help me get the word out. I want other women who suffer to know they're not alone.'

I feel weak but empowered.

In pain but now positive.

I wear yellow and I spray.

The sunflowers bloom and meander up my wall like tentacles from the Endobitch.

I share the growth each day on social media -and the first EndoWall is born.

The list of women lengthens. They ask for their names on the solitary black bricks nestled amongst nine yellow bricks.

Not just women from the UK but from Australia, South Africa, Canada, the USA. Argentina, France, Germany, Scandinavia...to name a few.

We're no longer merging with the crowd but standing up, standing out.

And shouting.

Shouting to be believed, helped, diagnosed, treated and most of all for research into why?!

Why?

What is the cause?

What is the cure?

Why is nobody listening?

Now we have a sisterhood. A support group.

We can share our stories. Give comfort and care. Just be there.
We are not alone.

In a year I have added 450 names to the first EndoWall.

450 names from the 176 million women worldwide.

Plus their partners, mothers, sisters, friends. All are affected. It's life-changing. Debilitating.

Endometriosis is a thief.

It steals days and months.

It steals years of our lives.

But we are not alone, and we are Warriors.

Even if we can't get the help we need in our own lifetimes, we've come together to start a movement to Raise Endo Awareness to help millions of women from future generations.

We want to help them.

Do you?

EndoWall 2 is on its way.

I just need permission for the next location …any ideas?

If you have a wall - just call.

You know how to find me!

Jaimee Rae McCormack and Laura Mccormack-Long
June 2018

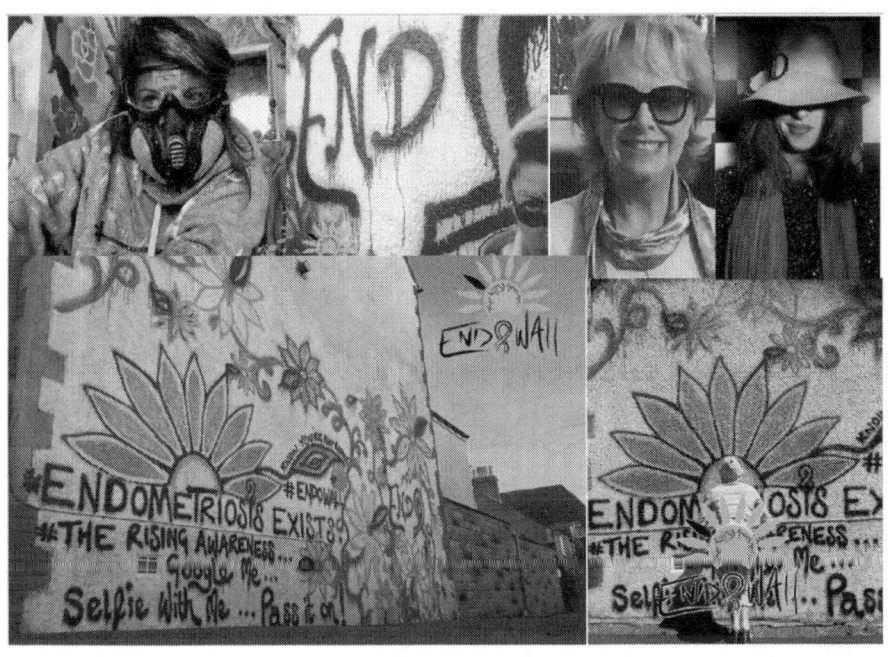

"We spend years of our life trying to convince doctors we are in pain and genuinely ill. Only to be given poor treatment that leads to misdiagnosis, pointless surgeries, trauma, infertility, depression, anxiety, physical, mental, emotional, spiritual and financial devastation. and so much more."

– *Imogene McClain*

TWENTY TWO

Imogene McClain, Iowa

I'm not a bitch. Endometriosis is a bitch.

Confessions by Imogene McClain

I find myself to have become a very literal person. One who can also appreciate metaphorical expressions. I do many things. I am a counselor, a performer, writer, singer, trainer, and a bunch of other certified things on official pieces of paper that will make me look less than humble. And certainly "not sick enough" to accomplish all that I have. I will come back to that.

I am writing this piece under my pen name, Imogene McClain, but the photos provided with my written contribution and personal testimony are me. I owe it to my endo sisters to explain why I am writing under a pen name at this time. I am simply living off the grid and taking much overdue self care. Nonetheless, I am telling my story. I am showing my face. I stand with my endo sisters.

I am going to share with you parts of my personal story and battle with the disease, Some facts and my own opinions as well. You do not have to agree with my opinions. But you cannot argue with the facts. So, before you continue reading, make sure you know the difference between a fact and an opinion. You will find yourself free of a lot of manipulation and cognitive distortions with just this simple acknowledgement and opportunity to self educate.

A large part of my identity is being a writer, so, of course, I implement metaphors. I have found metaphors are some of my favorite ways to explain to anyone who is not living with endometriosis, is often the most creative way to explain the misery and doom of endometriosis. Which to be clear are symptoms of the disease. No one chooses this misery and doom. Let's break down misery and doom.

One of the symptoms of endometriosis is excruciating, debilitating pain. The disease is taboo and on average it takes a woman 7-10 years to obtain diagnosis. In fact, the majority of women with endometriosis are not taken seriously and dismissed. We are told we are "over-reacting", being "over dramatic", that our pain is "normal."

Consequently, through these consistent dismissals, many of us are made to feel like we deserve it. Some even do believe that. I have met women that truly believe periods are supposed to be the most painful part of being a woman and the only way to cope is to accept it. Let me say that again. Accept it.

Not acknowledge that it is a disease that needs treatment or even deserves adequate research that could lead to a cure. But accept it and therefore accept suffering and despair. They even quoted some scripture to me about it. I held back my eye roll. That time anyway.

Can you imagine such despairing, relentless pain and then being told, and I quote, "it is just part of being a woman? Accept it. Get over it!" Spoken to me and millions of women from medical professionals desperately seeking answers.

I share this next experience with heavy resentment and anger I am still trying to reconcile in myself over twenty years later. After one of my surgeries, my doctor came in to explain he accidentally scraped my abdomen during the laproscopy. "But not to worry," as he oddly sensually massaged the scrape on my abdomen that a band aid and some neosporin would treat in a few days. He boldly continued after this offbeat, undesired caressing, "you are still very sexy."

This was said in the presence of my fiance at the time as I was barely coming out of the anesthesia, I think if I had not felt dazed, weak and still kind of asleep, I would have punched him in the face, if I am being honest. I tell you I sat straight up in the hospital bed with all my might and covered myself up from where he lifted my hospital gown to expose the scrape I barely noticed, that I wouldn't even describe as a wound, and said, "why don't you just get the fuck out of here?" I sat there in silence with my fiance as my doctor eerily took his time exiting my room while we were still wondering what in the actual fuck just happened.

He returned about twenty minutes later. I wasn't sure if he was going to ask me on a date, disrobe me, or actually review the photos from my surgery I saw him holding. I felt sick as he sat on my hospital bedside unnecessarily, but felt obligated to allow it if he were going to finally review and discuss the findings of my surgery I was so desperate to see.

Finally, he begins showing me photos from my laparoscopy which had evident, visible endometriosis everywhere. His next comment, "Not really sure what this is we are seeing, but you look so healthy. You certainly don't look sick. You are in really good shape. A beautiful woman. I wouldn't worry about this."

To make a long story short, I spent two more years jumping through what I am certain were made up intentional procedures to get those surgical photos and medical records. Once I had them, I found another doctor, did another surgery and she came right in and said, "You absolutely have endometriosis. I have also compared the photos from your last surgery and unfortunately your condition has worsened."

It is such a strange feeling when someone gives you an accurate diagnosis, tells you that you are not crazy, your pain is real and then you also have to acknowledge there is no cure. You are so grateful, so relieved to finally have some tell you what is really going on and it is a real disease and then devastated knowing you are going to fight this battle for the rest of your life.

To make a very long and sad story short, I had at least five more surgeries in a four year time span. And me being the workaholic I became, as a way to cope in unhealthy denial of my disease; after each surgery, I got up, got dressed and went straight back to work. I did not realize at the time that my pain tolerance had built quite high. I didn't have these super power coping strategies I convinced myself of afterall. Years and years of medical negligence and medical dismissals of my disease conditioned my body to tolerate insane amounts of pain.

I would work out for three to four hours at a time, run ten to fifteen miles at least six times a week. All while maintaining a 60 to 75 hour work week. Anything to distract myself from my reality. Or waste anymore time trying to find anyone who knew how to help me, because I was conditioned for the same disappointing dismissals. So, I avoided them and worked harder on telling lies to myself that I was coping just fine.

I can't tell you how many surgeries I have had or how many doctors I have seen. But I promise you that you cannot propose a treatment I have not tried. I tried risky treatments that left with me with irreparable consequences physically. I was willing to do anything to stop the pain, only to find myself trading one set of problems for another and getting no relief. And a shit ton of more problems.

Then inevitably finding my desperate self feeling more pathetic than ever with another medical professional asking me to explain my pain on a scale of one to ten. Having to rely on explaining to someone on this scale of "one to ten" the amount of pain I am experiencing isn't just a trigger, it limits my vocabulary to numbers and these numbers are not accurate when trying to explain to a medical professional that you have built such a high tolerance for pain, you no longer know where you fall on a scale of one to fucking ten. How about I explain all my symptoms and you tell me as a doctor where I fall on your scale of one to ten?

I get very irritated when people call endometriosis an invisible disease. I declare and argue that this is absolutely not an invisible disease. Endometriosis is clearly visible through a laparoscopy and certainly was in all of mine. This disease has been labeled and described as invisible, but the truth is it is the negligence and procrastination of diagnostic surgery that defines this as invisible, creating and contributing to more terminology that inaccurately describes this disease. Not only is endometriosis seen when treated by a surgeon who is educated and trained to do the correct procedures, endometriosis symptoms are so blatantly obvious.

We spend years of our life trying to convince doctors we are in pain and genuinely ill. Only to be given poor treatment that leads to misdiagnosis, pointless surgeries, trauma, infertility, depression, anxiety, physical, mental, emotional, spiritual and financial devastation. and so much more.

These women find it difficult to even obtain education or stable employment.

These women go through multiple surgeries year after year to continue to remove endometriosis that returns for so many women, no matter what they do.

Forced to live in agony. These women, by the way, there are 176 million of them worldwide, and counting. Wrap your mind around that for just one second. If all the women with endometriosis formed their own country, it would be the eighth largest. Can we just get real for a second folks? Would that be invisible on a map? If one in ten people (men and/or women) were in this much pain, requiring so much surgery and causing common cases of infertility with such a disease, it would be labeled an epidemic.

Fact: Endometriosis is as common as asthma and diabetes.

Fact: Endometriosis has no cure.

Fact: Hysterectomies do not cure Endometriosis.

Fact: Having a child doesn't either and another fact, not all women want children. We are suggested to have them anyway in an attempt to alleviate our symptoms and miraculously cure ourselves. Even though we already covered actually there is no cure.

Fact: Endometriosis has no known cause.

Fact: I have lived with endometriosis for over two decades. I fucking hate it. None of this is invisible.

Furthermore, people need to stop saying that talking about menstruation is gross or inappropriate. It's part of being a woman.

When people refuse to listen to these conversations, that also makes women invisible. The disease isn't invisible, our willingness to listen to women discuss their concerns is becoming invisible. When we as a society are willing to listen to women and celebrate them, value them, advocate for them, they will be empowered, heard, believed and taken seriously. An empowered woman who has been seen, heard, believed is a loyal woman.

We build strong women when we give them deserved and necessary validation. I have found a woman who is unconditionally loved by just one individual creates far more power than the conditioning of other women dependent on their rage to survive. In love, we thrive. In fear, we survive. I just don't know if I have it in me to survive one more thing.

Guaranteed you know someone with endometriosis. And guaranteed they need you.

Like I said, I find myself to have become a very literal person. One who can also appreciate metaphorical expressions. Perhaps, because this seems to be the only way to explain to friends, family and medical professionals the anguish of that dirty six syllable word no one seems to have heard of: ENDOMETRIOSIS.

For example, "you know, it's like someone inserting tiny ninjas into your uterus and carving their names with a machete on the lining of your intestines just because they can. Then having flesh eating reptiles sitting down for a picnic on your ovaries in fear an alligator is going to burst out of your vagina."

It's like trying to convince someone in a white lab coat (also known as the cloak of required, automatic trust and respect when worn) that your pain is so real and so agonizing, then dismiss your 'phantom" pain that all women just go through and "mansplain" that the emergency room is for emergencies as they draw you a map to the nearest Walgreens so that you can treat your childbirth pains with midol.

I have lived with the chronic pain of endometriosis for so long, I sometimes think I have lost my sense of humor. Along with my sense of humor, as my disease has progressed, I have lost time for hobbies. I lost interest in my hobbies and became obsessed and determined to find anyone who knew what was happening in my body.

I especially despise crude jokes about women and "aunt flow" jokes. I dare not try to explain or discuss my disease anymore, because I cannot find it in me to hear some ignorant joke or be asked the same questions, followed up with at least three remedies that cured their toe fungus. Because somehow toe fungus and endometriosis are comparable.

For over twenty-two years, I have lived this hell. The jokes just aren't funny. They never were.

I was fed up with dumb period jokes and PMS jokes before I heard the carelessness of them delivered on late night talk shows by men. At 16 years old, I couldn't relate to my female peers who found relief in their menstrual cycle with a tylenol and a chocolate bar. Even unsolicited insinuations slipping out of the mouths of other women, young, old and in between, began a series of quite literally trying everything from sleeping with my legs over my head to walking nearly twenty miles a day.

I lived in a lonely world of bizarre advice that concluded with the manipulative acceptance of, "it's just part of being a woman," "We all get cramps," "Your pain tolerance is low," or "have a baby, it really worked for me."

I was 13 years old when I got this inappropriate advice.

Oh, my story is complicated one, but no less complicated than millions of women worldwide who all have a disease called endometriosis that is as common as asthma and diabetes.

This is only one story that should shake you to your bones and motivate you off your ass to do something prolific. My personal experience and history tells me permisticially you won't. No one will. And the ones who are motivated enough to do something are too sick to. But so long as the word hope exists in our language, I will try. And in that hope, I just live with it. To be clear, I live with it. I do not accept it. I just live with it. There is no choice.

There are multiple surgeries. Lost friendships. Lost relationships. Lots of people "shoulding" all over you. "You should try this organic diet! You should try this new surgery! You should meet my cousin Beth! She has had two babies now and pain free, you should..."

You should shut the fuck up.

Listen, any woman living with endometriosis, we have done it all. We are so full of "should," that's why we can't even pretend to listen to the next piece of "should" that comes out of your mouth. You contribute to my metaphorical constipation when you fill me up with so much "should."

I live with so much humiliation. Even in my own marriage. My disease has been slandered and exploited online. And with all the energy I used to fight my disease, I had no energy to understand or confront my husband for using my disease to get online and witness him detail my struggles to cam girls under the excuse and hidden identity declaring he "cant have sex with my wife because of her endometriosis".

To be clear, this was not a symptom I had, but one of the excuses he used to continue this behavior for multiple years. An exaggeration in order to get pity to tip these girls less. Then faced with the dilemma if I do not "forgive" him, I am not the gracious woman he or I identify as and expected to be. But that's another tale of misery and doom. And I will face it in my own time and space.

Maybe I am just a woman fed up with bad behavior and think that it is more than fair that our society start seriously finding accurate treatment or a cure for a disease as common as asthma and diabetes.

Here in my writing would be a perfect time to bring up if this disease occured in men, there would be a cure.

We all know that. So, I will save my breath.

I have lost count of how many surgeries I have had. But I would rather talk about the symptoms of this disease. Chronic depression, ungodly fatigue, cramping that feels like labor pains, anxiety, inability to stabilize employment and education, have children in many cases and the unbearable loneliness and isolation. These are only a few of the symptoms.

I secretly cringe when I hear one of my female companions say, "Oh damn I just started my period, do you have a Midol?" When I start my period, I fall to my knees and as an atheist, in my desperation, I beg God for mercy. This pleading goes on for days. Man, when I get in that desperate state, I have never wanted to believe in a miracle more and know what hope and faith feel like again. Sweating. Vomiting. Screaming in absolute terror and agony on the bathroom floor with excessive bleeding.

And more advice of, "You know, just because you are having your period, doesn't give you the right to make the rest of us miserable with your crying and bad attitude."

I wish I knew what it was like to choose a bad attitude. I need to make this very clear. I have a great attitude. I have a very painful disease.

Do not measure my character when I am in the fetal position on the floor of my bathroom in my own vomit crying uncontrollably in anguish and then tell me I am choosing to have a bad attitude about it.

First of all, no one is asking you to stand outside the bathroom door while I cry and scream and fight with all of our might to not lose hope. In fact, it just contributes to the humiliation and unbearable embarrassment.

Support and advocacy and really caring for someone is done with empathy and kindness. If my "attitude" gets measured when I am symptomatic and someone decides I am choosing that pain and those responses, they are the problem 100% of the time. Symptoms are a response to a disease. You do not choose them. But I tell you what, I feel an expectation to pretend they are not there.

I wish I knew what attitude to choose while I am in the fetal position, dehydrated, dry heaving so hard I have tunnel vision and my ears are ringing, all while experiencing the cramping of labor contractions. To choose to not cry uncontrollably in anguish so that those who want to support me can do so much easier. Believe me, I would shut it off if I could. You have a choice I do not have. To shut down your ignorant, unsolicited, uneducated, insensitive advice. And I demand that you do.

You would not say to a woman in labor, "You have no right to cry and scream like that. You need to find another way to express your pain in a way that does not disturb others."

Let me remind you again that endometriosis is a lonely disease. We do not request company in order to salvage the little humility and dignity we have left. The hypocrisy is that your judgements and unrealistic expectations of how I manage my disease and symptoms are what I call not just a bad attitude, but being a bad person. Don't project your bad attitude and nasty character and relate it to my disease.

You don't have a disease. You need a character makeover.

As the decades go by, your pain tolerance increases and your support system decreases. You learn to just shut up. Everyone around you is so sick of you because you didn't take their advice, yet they refuse to acknowledge that taking their advice most certainly would only have made you sicker. Then bitter. And lonelier as that person too soon leaves your life. Leaving all the blame with you when you know damn well the only one to blame is that bitch endometriosis.

You learn to be silent because when you're crying and legitimately, righteously angry about these skin and bones you are stuck in, you are told from someone who lives free of chronic pain and disease in their own skin, "Being cranky and complaining about your pain only reflects on your character."

Let me tell you something about my character. I know who I am. I know I am a good person who has a disease that turned my life upside down. It didn't change me. It changed my responses. I am adapting to a world that has no cure for my disease. And I am doing the best I can.

I am not going to pretend it is not there nor am I going to pretend I am happy I have this disease. Stop telling me I have something to learn from this. Because I am leaning every single day to be more gracious and patient with myself. I refuse to be dismissed any longer and am dismissing those who are giving horrible advice, engaging in blatant medical negligence and malpractice and taking my power back. Because I am not alone.

We outnumber those who have dismissed us by millions. Don't forget that number. 176 million women. And counting.

I am grieving so many things. I am grieving in my own space and time. I can't fight every day. You wouldn't ask someone who has been shot in the leg to walk a mile. So, no, I cannot smile every single day.

Sometimes I miss events I have been looking forward to for days, months, years. The worst part of missing these events with my loved ones, is often being shamed and sometimes even gaslighted because I am physically incapable of just "sucking it up". I am tired of pushing myself that hard. I have played multiple three to four hour-long performances as a singer even less than 24 hours after surgery. I did that three times! I have worked myself to exhaustion and I don't just deal with endometriosis in the serious way I need to and finally am.

I am a sexual assault survivor that also requires my attention, responsibility and intention to heal and recover. I love myself enough to do that.

Look, I am legitimately happy for people who live free of chronic pain and trauma. I am learning not to envy you. I am legitimately happy you do not have what I have. I'm not done fighting. If I were, I wouldn't be this fucking pissed off.

I do my best work when I am this angry and fed up. I am spending my time these days restoring years of pushing myself too hard. I am learning to be gentle and kind to myself. Taking the break I need. I will be back. Healed. And ready with good energy, balance, well rested, and determination that never left me. I know 176 million other women who feel the same way.

Give us your advocacy, energy and support. Really hear us. Be on the right side of history. Believe me, it is the hope and faith I dream of when I want to believe in miracles.

There are still an alarming amount of women who will not speak in fear of further mistreatment, public shaming or humiliation, and for some, even confessed prescription drug addiction due to their ongoing painful symptoms of endometriosis and continue to be seen by doctors who provide poor clinical oversight and care.

I have interviewed so many women with endometriosis and each woman's story is unique. The common factor is unnecessary suffering. Their confessions were crucial to bringing awareness to the poor clinical treatment giving to women suffering from endometriosis. Many women were also unable to participate due to crippling pain and chronic fatigue, disabling their ability to provide testimony even from their own home or by phone.

I honor the confidentiality of all women whom I have contacted or been contacted by over the years and in no way will reveal their identity or lead to the discovery of their identity. However, it is important to hear their struggles and to understand the seriousness of the disease.

There is great despair and great suffering for such a large group of women. Please hear them. Please listen. We want to tell you not just what it's like for us, but how endometriosis is affecting our entire society economically as well. Think of the millions of women with unlimited potential limited by this disease that could impact the world globally in so many ways if they could relieve their suffering. They belong, they are welcome and have so much to offer the world.

It turns out if you listen to women, believe them, and are not dismissive, you can learn a lot about them. Without dedicated, ongoing research to the crippling disease of endometriosis that leads to diagnosis, fair and ethical treatment and the public demanding such, we will continue to see a large group of women ignored and oppressed.

By now, I do hope you're concerned.

You've learned we are all impacted by this disease. We may have even reflected and after some soul searching, perhaps we silenced someone at some point. Here is what you can do. Talk about it. Be there. Demand research from the medical community. Fight with us. For a better life. Through the hard days. For a cure. For women. For peace. For less pain, the ending of needless suffering, more empathy and more understanding. To break the silence. To empower. To dry the tears. To take our hand. For a quality life.

You don't have to have endometriosis to be part of the army of women afflicted fighting for their rights to just live, be seen, be heard, and advocated for. 176 million women and counting are unable to obtain and maintain employment, missing educational opportunities, drowning in medical debt, isolated from social events, unable to provide for themselves and dependent on caretakers. Some are bed bound in excruciating pain battling depression, anxiety and some contemplating suicide. And some battling addiction too.

They need advocacy. They need support. They need help. They need you.

We speak politically and fight for equal pay for women in the workforce, a woman's right to choose, and free of sexism. We demand the removal of oppression and suppression with legislative action and activism, yet there is still a large group of women not being heard.

There are 176 million women and counting who are so ill they have not the opportunity, able body, or support to seek desired education, explore their potential and talents to secure that dream career in equal employment. Women are still suffering; impolied they're required to suffer because it's part of being a woman.

Women are being ignored and becoming more and more ill with this disease, because they are not believed and simple, prompt procedures can be done when symptoms are heard and not measured on a scale of one to ten.

To obtain a diagnosis, they are still taking nearly a decade to accomplish. They are silenced because their period "is supposed to be painful and miserable." Male and female doctors are committing these acts contributing to the suppression and oppression of women globally who are driven to silence, mental illness, drug and alcohol addiction, unemployment, poverty, as the result of ignorance and refusal to acknowledge a very common but also excruciating disease called endometriosis that impacts one in ten women.

Women all over the world are suffering, trapped in their own bodies missing opportunity, shamed by doctors and ignored in society.

It's a lonely disease. For so many reasons. Prolonged exposure to such horrific pain and trauma conditions a person. Drives them to insanity and has conditioned responses that are out of character and speaking from a dark place of desperateness. It's not easy being the caretaker for a woman with endometriosis. Their partners and families also suffer as there is no cure and few treatment options that are helpful.

These women have dreams, aspirations and hopes of having a family. But endometriosis for many women brings infertility with its luggage of consequences.

Women with endometriosis are known as the "flakes" who are inconsistent and can never keep plans when they are struck down with symptoms that immobilize them. It's difficult for friends and family to understand that having a period or ovulating can disable a woman to the point she cannot bring herself out of bed, much less attend a family gathering. And even worse, lack of employment and leaves her unable to provide for herself.

Lack of research on how homelessness affects women with endometriosis will only keep the public ignorant. We don't even know how many exact suicides in women were definitely due to endometriosis. It's clumped in there somewhere with depression. But the root of that depression is endometriosis for some who are suffering in despair.

I believe that there are good people in the world who do want to help. And they need research and facts so they can be educated. But first, we must believe women. We must see them and hear them. You are not going to get the data you need if you only accept a number between one and ten. You need it all.

Without awareness, research can't be accomplished. And we cannot teach awareness if we are not willing to believe women the first time. We still know too little still about endometriosis and how far the impact of the suffering reaches.

And if you still don't think it impacts you, I remind you to understand how this is contributing to our economy. There are able minded women desperate to relieve their pain to achieve appropriate education and employment. Talented, intelligent, incredible women who are "unemployable" all because of endometriosis. Economically speaking, this costs society millions of dollars annually in the United States. Women are unable to provide for themselves contributing to the workforce and our economy. Additionally, unable pay their medical bills that can include hormone treatment, multiple surgeries, exams, medication and more. Their caretakers miss work as well. And severe depression and anxiety are the result of these stressors.

It's a merciless disease. Not only are women told they are overreacting or over dramatic, their symptoms leave them begging and pleading for relief. But it never comes.

It's a taboo disease. No one likes a complainer. Especially a woman who is complaining. Aren't women already labeled complainers? After all, "it's just part of being a woman" and you know, women can't talk about their periods. That's totally gross and inappropriate.

But what if I need to leave work because I am bleeding through my clothes? What if I am in so much pain, I feel like I am having a child? Would you ask a woman in labor to stay at work? Would you tell her "this is part of being a woman." Would you ask her, "On a scale of one to ten, one being the least pain you ever felt and ten being the worst?

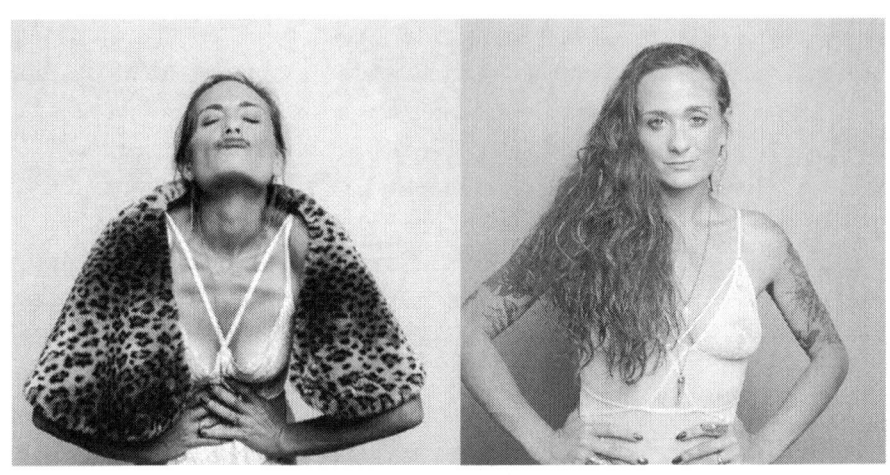

PHOTOGRAPHS BY MICHAEL WATSON

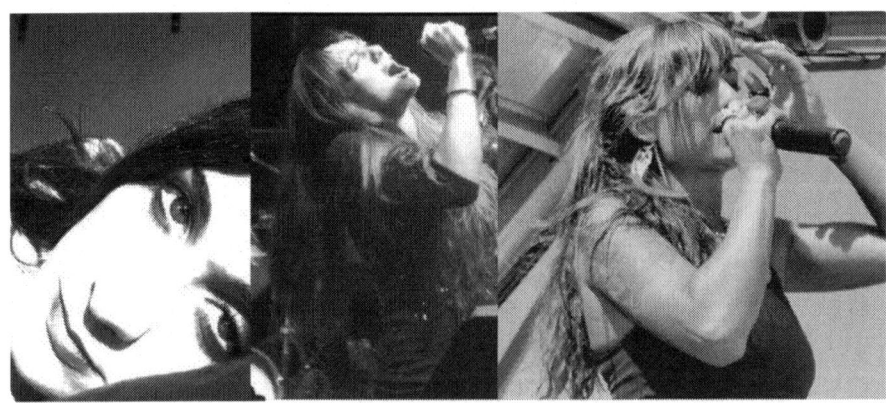

"The more I learn about the disease, the numerous injustices, healthcare inadequacies and concerns for conflicting interest among the stakeholders of the endometriosis community, the greater my passion for change becomes."

— Dr. Wendy Bingham, DPT

TWENTY THREE

Dr. Wendy Bingham (DPT), Washington

Everyone admired my tenacity to pursue and accomplish the goals and dreams I had. The ones I thought were my destiny, despite the odds. My goals and 'life's goals' apparently differ. 'Life' has its own plans for me, whether I want them or not.

…let's go back in time…

It doesn't make any sense. I got this pain that shows up once in a while. It's tucked up-and-under my ribs on the right side. The pain also feels like its 'inside my collarbone', kind of like dry-ice or an ice-cold steel pipe. A sensation that's so cold it feels hot. Every breath I take, the pain in my collarbone feels like its dancing with the pain up-under my ribs.

My doctor thinks it's a 'side-stitch'. Funny thing is, I get them on both sides. Not usually at the same time though. I don't know what it is, but it interferes with my ability to run with the cross-country team. It's my Senior year of high school. I have never been fast enough to make the Varsity Squad. But running is my opioid. Running provides a sense of freedom. Life in a broken home where alcohol has permeated the integrity of family and the inherent platform from which self-confidence emerges, running is my support system.

It's My Time. Setting crazy goals like, high mileage, rough terrain and variable altitude in ridiculous weather conditions is routine. Conquering, the unconquerable, drives me. Doing the impossible gives me self-worth; never the best at anything but never giving up. I run.

This year I had a lot of inconsistencies. For some reason, I have periods of time where it's hard to breath. It's like a workout just to catch my breath. The doctors thought I had asthma, but the preliminary tests in the doctor's office were inconclusive. My results have been different from each test session. One of the two episodes indicated I 'may' be 'borderline asthmatic'. Whatever that means. Nobody has given me inhalers or anything else to try.

The coach decided to have a run-off at the District Championships to determine which of us (my teammate or I) would fill the 8th and final slot for the State Championships. The District Championship was yesterday. I didn't race well. I won't be representing my school at the State Championships. What bothers me, is why.

That horrible pain crept up again during warm-ups. The harder I tried to run, the pain got stronger and spread. It travelled up my neck, jaw and even my ear. Normally when it happens I can 'run through it' by slowing down and patiently wait for it to subside. I did not have that luxury during a race. When I sped up, the pain got worse, and my breathing was all-over the place.

Have you tried running while you're ready to cry? It's awful. Being upset, I couldn't breathe correctly. I couldn't get enough air, so I would try to breath in harder and deeper, which only reinforced the pain. By the time the pain subsided I was too far behind to make a challenge. I congratulated my teammate. I didn't tell my coach. He's the type of coach who doesn't like to hear excuses.

…fast forward…

It's nice to return to England and be with my fiancé. My fiancé and I met while I spent a year abroad in college. I went home for a semester to complete my requirements for a Bachelor of Science. It's been about a year since I returned. It's really weird to be a patient in a hospital of a foreign country. Although I wrote a paper about the NHS in England and professional duties of Physiotherapists while at University on exchange, I currently work part-time in the Business Development Office of the new forming Trust, and volunteer one night a week as a 'candy striper' at the Lancaster Royal Infirmary delivering items to patients on the wards.

I never thought I would BE a patient on the wards I regularly visited. My care is wonderful. Unfortunately, it's the first of many journeys where the sources of my pains are not identified. My gastrointestinal system has been acting up more and more the past few years. I recently developed this severe right side, lower abdominal cramping and feeling of 'hot pokers'. The pain travelled right through me. I thought it was my appendix but it also felt like it travelled through my pelvic hip bone, and groin. Literally that same 'cold steel pipe' sensation I still get in my collarbone. It makes my right leg feel very weak, like 'jello' when I walk. Lots of tests but nothing found.

…fast forward…

My husband and I are back in America now. We spent the first year working temporary jobs. My husband accepted a position that relocated us across the country. After a year, I enrolled in graduate school for Physical Therapy. That hasn't kept me out of the ER. But. I'm still running. I've even done some marathons. I am no Greta Waitz or Joan Benoit Samuelson, but it's My Time.

There are no doctors who have figured out what my pains are from. The pains can't be anything serious or they would have figured it out by now. Besides, running is my opiate. It's what gives me tenacity. I need it. It's more important than the breathing problems, chest pains and all the gastrointestinal problems that keep getting worse.

I thought the mileage I run was the problem. You know, 'runners trots'. But it's crazy. I notice more and more that my tummy swells and the diarrhea is worse around my menstrual cycles. I assume it's just 'water weight' that normally happens during the premenstrual time. I look and feel like a water balloon. I've never asked my friends or compared my experiences. I assume its normal. That includes the more recent 'swing' the other direction I've been having: constipation. It does seem strange for a runner to regularly have constipation.

When I feel like a water balloon, it's very sensitive to touch my skin. I really hate tight clothing. Even more weird, when I swell up like a balloon, the right side of my stomach bulges more than the left. Then there's the groin pain. It spreads up my lower abdomen on the right. It feels like it travels straight through my sacrum (bone in back of pelvis). It makes my leg feel really heavy and hard to pick up. It's this deep ache. It comes and goes like all the others. I do notice it tends to be worse with my period. Of course. But. The chest pains. I hate them the most. They're getting worse. I don't like to complain about them because they usually last a few minutes to maybe, half an hour.

Sometimes the sharp pains come quick. Any movement or breathing, the pain 'immobilizes' me until it passes. I know they are pleural pains, (and like the other pains, always in the same spots). Per all of my doctors, it's considered a benign condition. What makes it worse, my body has become a barometer. I develop a diffuse deep ache in my chest, on the left side. It feels like I've been kicked by a horse.

The internet is still an 'infant'. There's no such thing as Smart Phones. I'm now a meteorologist able to detect storms approaching within half-an-hour. Who needs to read the forecast or look to the sky, the aches in my chest are fairly accurate at predictions.

…fast forward…

It's been nine months in my first position as a Physical Therapist. I love working in the Rehabilitation Hospital. The strangest thing happened. I was feeling extra-tired at the end of a long week (more than the usual working a physical job about 55 hours a week). It was the start of our Friday afternoon patient session. I was walking back from the cafeteria when I experienced a very hot, sharp stab in my left shoulder blade. It proceeded to send those familiar nerve pains up my neck, jaw and ear.

I immediately felt unwell and shaky. Unsure if I could safely handle my patients that afternoon, I chose to go home. I was very lethargic the rest of the weekend. I didn't exercise; in-fact, I hardly left the couch. I did manage to unload the dishwasher. But it was agony. Each time I bent to grab plates I felt 'bubbles' move down my back. When I returned upright, the bubbles travelled back up toward my neck followed by 'intense pain' atop my shoulder, neck and jaw.

It literally felt like I had a bowling ball sitting on my shoulder and could hardly turn my head in that direction. Each time I changed positions, the bubbles would move to the uppermost position, then after a short delay, the pain would reappear.

By Monday I still was not better. I struggled to make a flight of stairs and could hardly breath. I called into work and told them I seemed to have a 'bout of pleurisy that I can't shake'. So off to the doctor's office I went. It was revealed I had a Spontaneous Pneumothorax. It landed me in the hospital for 24 hours observation.

Due to the size of the collapse, it was borderline to treat with a chest tube or observation with supplemental O2. I will tell you; I did not sleep much that night. Between the air in my chest making audible 'clicking' sounds with my heartbeat, and the chest tube tray in view at my bedside (as a 'just-in-case'), was not a fun experience. Little did I know, it was just the beginning.

On my return to work, a respiratory therapist I work with approached me. He too had suffered numerous spontaneous pneumothoraxes that were eventually diagnoses as 'Primary Spontaneous Pneumothorax'. His condition resolved with a thoracotomy to remove the blebs from his lung.

Now remember, these are the days before 'Internet' and instant access to abundant information doesn't exist. In our conversation, and I will NEVER FORGET this, "Make sure they (lung collapse(s)) don't align with your periods." Well, actually, now that he mentioned it; I started my period Saturday morning after the incident Friday afternoon at work. Seeing his scar, I thought, how absurd that a lung problem could be related to my menstrual cycles. Remember, internet is an infant. Not only is Thoracic Endometriosis and Catamenial Pneumothorax barely recognized entities in the new millennium, even less information was available about the condition and how to treat it at the time of these events in my life.

To an extent, I was also in denial. To see my co-worker's full thoracotomy scar was overwhelming. If I ignored and denied any possibility that my 'popping' lung and periods were related, I wouldn't need to endure something like that. So, over the years, no matter where my conscious degree of 'acceptance' was, guess who paid much closer attention to the relationship between my periods and symptoms I experienced? Yep. Our conversation remained in my memory. Still, I run.

...pause from the timeline...temporal pattern of symptoms over the year.

What transpired over the years? In the first few years after the first documented spontaneous pneumothorax, during the week prior to menses, symptoms would rebuild, nearly every month before menses. Symptoms were most intense the day before my cycle then quickly subside after my periods started. (chest pains, fluctuations in my breathing, bowel and bladder changes and even intimacy concerns).

Over the years, the peak intensity of symptoms moved from the day before my period to Day One of my menses. In the final months/year prior to excision surgery the culmination of scapular stabbing, trickling liquid in my chest and nerve pain peaking 10 minutes prior to my menstrual cycle starting! The anxiety, every month, waiting for the buildup, hoping it would skip a month, or better yet, never return. It was dreadful.

Adding injury to insult, despite the detail and clarity of my symptoms, history and timeline association, not a single physician associated the events, perceived the magnitude of what I experienced or that a relationship existed between my menstrual cycle and the other concerns. The first 'I believe you', began the final two years of a thirty-year journey without a diagnosis. Long after considerable damage had been done.

Anxiety built every month. Over the years, the episodic periods grew into a continuous presence of symptoms present through the entire month. Symptoms did rise and fall, with a subpeak at ovulation, a temporary wane the following week, then a greater rise and peak on the first day of my periods.

There are countless times I have been out in public when the peak arrived. I would briefly lose connection to my surrounding environment. My focus automatically drawn inward. A feeling my body was trying to shut down, conserve energy and protect itself from potential harm by limiting available energy to continue activity and any ability I made to 'ignore' the pains that I had, so routinely for many years. My legs get weak, I feel the world closing in darkness. It's hard to understand voices around me. The only thing I can do is focus on the sensations and keep breathing. I feel my eyes opening wider, trying to ensure I do not pass out.

Many times I wish I could pass out before the sequela develops and wake up after the peak passed. However, the ability to feel the sensations imparted reality that I was still awake and 'present'. Either scenario, not having control, particularly out in public is a fear many of us have. Still, I run.

...Fast forward...

Our one and only child has arrived in the world. With elation comes exhaustion. I was actually excited for ONE benefit of nursing after childbirth; absence of a monthly period. Not!

In actual fact, my menstrual cycle returned 3 months postpartum. Even worse, a BIG Pneumothorax returned the day before my period restarted. This time the Chest Tube became a temporary accessory. Attempts to breastfeed on the involved side have not been successful from that point. Ouch, ouch, ouch.

The guilt remains with me that I could not provide one of the most important starts for my child. The body of some mother's are able to compensate. When one 'faucet' becomes 'out of order', the other 'faucet' produces more to meet their baby's needs. Supplemental formula became part of our feeding routine.

...fast forward one month...

Twenty eight days after the last pneumothorax, and cursed return of my menstrual cycle, another pneumothorax. I am now four months postpartum.

Did the thoracic surgeon recognize the association with my cycles? No. However, repetitiveness was acknowledged and an exploratory surgery was offered again. I declined. Had our situation been different, I may have elected for the procedure. At the time, would the surgeon have known what to look for? My husband recently became redundant from his employer of eight years. We had a three month-old infant and a mortgage. The thought of massive medical debt was greater than either my husband or I could grasp.

Over the next few years I continued to have regular episodes of pain. Sometimes I could feel my lung 'clunking around' inside my chest, bumping the walls of my ribcage when I changed positions.

Summers were awful. Dependent upon timing to my monthly cycle, entering air-conditioned buildings from the hot air outside created a sensation of 'fireworks' launching inside of my chest. Literally, hundreds of tiny icepicks in my chest accompanied by involuntary muscle contractions that made me 'grunt'. Think of this: All these pains occurring – fight or flight mode to get out of the building as fast as possible; the faster I moved the worse the pain! These same circumstances waxed and waned over years. Restaurants, grocery stores, movie theatres, homes of friends and family etc. Still, I ran.

…fast forward…

We moved cross-country again. Prior to moving, I worked on-call at the rehabilitation hospital and completed my transitional Doctorate of Physical Therapy (tDPT). I noticed my fatigue was getting stronger and stronger the past few years. Fatigue, not like I simply got tired earlier. Fatigue like, everything I did seemed to require higher levels of energy and longer periods to recover. Instead of feeling refreshed after a solid night's rest, I would awake with the sensation I never slept.

I had been to the ER for unexplained right lower quadrant pain and IBS-like symptoms a few times. One time, I was convinced I had appendicitis after performing the 'Bounce Home Test' on myself at home (in standing you rise up on your toes then drop your weight onto your heels. If pain reproduces and centers at McBurney's Point – a specific spot on the abdomen, its highly probable for appendicitis.) Three attempts, all three positive.

A long night in the ER. No diagnosis. This enquire led me on a journey toward my first colonoscopy. Oh, how pleasant. Results-normal.

Conclusion, the 'garbage can' diagnosis of 'Irritable Bowel Syndrome (IBS)' was given. Since our last move, I've become progressively more exhausted. I thought I knew what exhausted was. This is different. This is, all…the…time. The only way I can describe the sensation: carrying 1,000 pounds on my back (physically), just finished my Physical Therapist Licensure examination (mentally), and my best friend suddenly passed away (emotionally). All day, every day. No rest or length of sleep makes an impact.

...fast forward...

Our son is in middle school. A lot of stressful situations. Emotional stress definitely exacerbates the fatigue and cycle. The chest pains are getting worse. The bowels, on day one of my menses – I dread. Searing pain deep inside with each bowel movement (honey them ain't hemorrhoids either!). The days of alternating diarrhea and constipation no longer occur. Now, continuous constipation.

All...the...time.

I haven't been able to sit at 90 degrees to eat or work at computer. I can hardly eat, even small meals. I feel full easily, sometimes vomit after meals and sleep 14 hours every day (at the minimum) feeling like I never went to bed. Sleep is not 'replenishing'. I felt like I could pass out just standing in the kitchen preparing a meal. A 'run' has become a 'plod'. The 'plod' has dwindled to 20 minutes a few times a week.

Still, I run.

My neighbor, who is the same age as me, and seems fit-as-a-fiddle, was just diagnosed with a rare form of cancer. She has a husband and three children. This news has kept me up at night. Over the past six months or so, the pain in my right lower abdomen is getting a lot worse, it's that pain I always get at ovulation. It's never been this bad. Now it's all the time, but hottest before my period and keeps me awake at night.

I hate seeing a gyn. In fact, I haven't seen one in about 4 yrs. The pelvic exam is uncomfortable and the pap smear burns like a bee sting.

I have avoided the regular doctor the past few years. In part, the clinic I attend, shuffles doctors through so fast I never have the same one twice. I never feel like I am never taken seriously by doctors. I find it strange, perhaps because I am a medical provider myself. Is this normal? Do women who aren't medical providers feel the same way? Their body language, words and lack of recommendation continues to give me the sense that 'it's not that bad'.

Gee, even though I am getting older, should I have these pains keep recurring and progressing? Is it normal to have lung collapses that just occur? Is it normal to have fatigue THIS bad? Wow, if it is, I can't imagine how I'm going to survive my golden years. I am getting really frustrated. My husband mentioned a doctor in town he just started seeing. I am going to give it a try.

I met my new doctor. I'm hopeful. He is a Doctor of Osteopathy. I've worked with many DO's in rehab and am comfortable speaking with them. I am happy about this. My anxiety every time I enter a doctor's office to explain my problems, I start talking faster and sometimes go blank trying to find words. I am so afraid of being dismissed and having tests that come back normal. All my life I never gave up with anything I wanted to do. I pushed myself through numerous marathons and earned a Doctorate degree. Am I really imagining it's 'all in my head'? Am I reacting to a paper cut like it's a limb amputation?

At my first visit with the DO, I mentioned the severe fatigue to start the conversation and discussed the right lower abdominal concerns. I also mentioned my upcoming appt with a Gynecologist. My first impression: he's a good listener.

He seems to prefer a partnership with his patients, not the traditional paternal doctor-patient relationship. I had blood tests and, after listening to my heart, the nurse collected an EKG. A few abnormalities were found on the EKG. Although my resting heart rate of 38-42 beats-per-minute is normal for me, he referred me to a cardiologist for some minor atypical readings.

My new doctor mentioned, as we age, sometimes what was a normal heart rate for you when you are more active may become a concern as we age. He thinks maybe this contributed to the heavy fatigue I am experiencing. My appointment with the Cardiologist is still a few weeks away so off, after I meet with the new gynecologist.

My visit with the new Gynecologist only lasted 15 minutes. I explained my concerns to her. She did a basic pelvic exam (a pelvic exam that, as I sit here writing this, now I know significantly lacked thoroughness.) This was followed by "well you are getting older and it's probably just the changes. But let's get an ultrasound and check everything out." OK. She made it sound like its' no big deal. I kind of feel like a wimp. To me, the pain I have seems more than just 'getting older', but she says its "normal."

Another day, another doctor. I met the Cardiologist today. I don't like him. From the minute he walked into the room my perception was, 'this guy thinks I am a middle-aged woman with high anxiety that does not need to be here'. My gut feeling was confirmed by our conversation.

I mentioned my background as a very athletic woman who has had some respiratory concerns on and off over the years, a documented heart murmur due to the athlete's heart from years of running. I also mentioned the familial cardiac history in my family. I spoke about the degree of exhaustion and inability to even 'jog' due to fatigue, shortness of breath and nerve pains.

Here is the 'kicker' ... He looked directly at me and asked "If you were asked to run an 8-minute mile, do you think you could do it?" I replied 'No'. He asked me again. I was a bit more uncomfortable the second time but still replied 'No'. When he asked me the same question a third time ... I began counting with my fingers, firmly grasping the underside of my chair to keep track.

The more times he asked me, my anxiety continued to rise and self-doubt that my concern was not serious. I went through the fingers of my right hand twice. The eighth time he asked the same question (yep!), I finally replied 'Yes, I think I could'.

I find his actions were very unprofessional. At the consultation with him I was vulnerable. I was exhausted, been shuffled around without answers from doctors and oft felt dismissed of my concerns. I could not articulate at the time how I felt, being inappropriately treated, desperate for someone to believe me and help me. Looking back, I feel he used his position of authority and decision making along with a bias of women as hysterically amplifying their symptoms of non-emergent, often anxiety driven symptoms for benign conditions.

The cardiologist consultation concluded with him stating that, based upon my age and family history a treadmill stress test is appropriate to detect any abnormalities. Really? Was the repetitive, same question necessary? What purpose did it serve?

Tomorrow is my Stress Test. It's been a long time since I 'jogged'. I think I should get my body into a rhythm so I can push as hard as I can to figure out what is wrong. THAT damn pain is back again. Today, it's on the right side up and under my ribs. Its shooting into my collarbone, jaw and ear. I can't even 'plod' a lap around the neighborhood ... and it's STILL there. The air is super thick and a lot of effort to breathe in. I can't get enough air.

That attempt to jog sucked. I've been sitting here on the coach for a few minutes after getting back to the house. THAT pain is still there.

Here comes the 'shaky' sensation. It feels dark in the house.

That gross sensation of liquid trickling down inside my chest (behind my left breast). The stabbing sensations in my chest and shoulder blade. Jason, from Friday the 13th has arrived.

The last thing ... nerve pain up the left side of my neck, now matching the right side. My ears hurt.

Wait.

Here it comes.

Yep, my period has arrived.

It's been five days since the Stress Test. I'm not feeling very well. I had a scare that day. I felt embarrassed to mention it at the time it was happening.

The technicians did not seem concerned with any findings so it can't be anything very bad, despite how awful I feel.

…let me take you back…

I ran really hard. They kept pushing me to reach the projected maximum heart rate. I couldn't get my heart rate that high. Even I knew that a starting heart rate of 38-42 bpm was not going to reach an age set limit based upon normal resting rates. Of course, after the test they clarified that my resting rate and heart size may have been factors (uh, yeah). That wasn't the concern. During the treadmill testing, THAT pain and 'trickle' started up again. But, it was only located in the chest. I did not experience any nerve pain travelling up into my neck, jaw and ear.

They made a note of it at the corresponding time of EKG trace. During the first five minute recovery phase, while lying flat, immediately at the end of the run, the same 'trickle and THAT focal point pain reappeared. After a full 20 minutes I was able to get up and return to the changing rooms. I did not feel well and was 'shaky'. I mentioned this to the technician. He stated that the adrenaline can sometimes make people feel 'a bit off' for a while.

I changed my clothes and headed out through the waiting room. I stopped. I still really did not feel well. Something wasn't right. I have done numerous strenuous athletic activities but this is different. I honestly didn't know what to do. I did not want to make a scene. My husband is out of town, my son is in school. I can't have anything go wrong anyway.

My brain returned to the default mentality after years of uncorroborated explanation for my concerns, 'if it was serious they would have detected something' and self-esteem kept me from pursuing help.

I got in my car, proceeded to the freeway. That unwell feeling became a hot, brittle sensation across my entire chest. Distracted and anxious, I didn't realize I was travelling the wrong direction on the freeway to get home (not the wrong way of traffic – just wrong direction to get home). I pulled off the freeway and took the backroad home. In fact, I drove directly past my primary care doctor's office. I nearly stopped. I was really scared something was wrong. My anxiety over dismissal and no findings made me drive straight past the office.

It's five days later. Today is the first since the Stress Test I am able to get up from the sofa. The sofa I have slept on and rarely moved from the past 4 days. The pleurisy pains and gurgling have been relentless. Simply trying to breath or get up to use the bathroom has been met by the firing squad in my chest. I followed up with my primary care doctor today. Of course he's upset with me.

Especially after I finally disclosed my history of pneumothoraxes and cyclical chest pains that coincide my periods. Knowing this, he wants me to visit a thoracic surgeon. Why didn't I report these issues before to my new DO? Trust, brain fog and history of dismissal without answers, its presence became part of my life and had to accept it.

Life is no longer about thriving. Life is about surviving.

I finally recovered from the pleural pains induced from the stress test. It only took twelve days! But now, I am here having my Pelvic Ultrasound. I am so exhausted. The imaging technician is poking around my right ovary. I'm not a 'happy camper'. The radiologist is showing me a complex cyst on my Right ovary. Honestly, I'm so exhausted. It can't be anything more concerning that what I have just gone through.

I lay there, listening, concerned, but too numb from the recent events to think of and articulate some of the unusual events that have transpired recently. He says I should get it, (the complex cyst), out very soon. He also noticed my endometrium is abnormally thick for the time of my menstrual cycle. A lot of prior ultrasound reports over the years have the same findings but no one has ever discussed these or asked me questions. That right ovary is also, always the sore one, especially during ovulation (mid-month). The term 'mittelschmerz' comes to thought.

My appointment with the thoracic surgeon is coming up. You won't believe this. I was standing in the kitchen preparing dinner while my husband and son were playing soccer in the backyard. I wave of nausea and shakiness came over me. I felt, what I knew, to be the cyst on my ovary, rupture. There went dinner.

I heard so many stories of ruptured cysts but never to my knowledge, experienced one. Everyone I spoke to said a trip to the ER and $250 copay isn't worth it. They simply send you home.

My first consultation with a thoracic surgeon since my son was born, over a decade ago. Her first words to me as she entered the room "You don't have an immediate concern, what can I do for you?" All spoken while dropping my chart on the desk, not even turning to make eye contact.

My hope already gone. My heart sank. I wanted to cry.

I don't cry. I can't cry – I'm suppose to be a fighter. I did not get this far in life without fighting for everything. I felt insignificant, tiny. What I feel, my fears and life goal must not be important. How can I articulate how severe the symptoms have become? How can I articulate that I can't function anymore?

I had been waiting for what felt like forever, hardly able to sit upright in the chair for her to enter that room. All the while, my heart beating in my chest and perspiration flowing. Following her grand entrance and comment, I turned and grabbed my notes next to me; copies of the body diagrams and calendar journal of my menstrual cycle that detailed all associated symptoms. My voice was already quivering. My head swirled. Why bother to try to explain? She won't believe you. She will think you are crazy. She will tell you 'It's too rare'.

Evidently, my anxiety to tell her and past experiences of dismissal was interpreted by her as 'you seem to be very anxious. It is a good idea to talk to your primary care doctor about something to help with the anxiety.' She then suggested that my symptoms be managed as such "at your age, you don't need a period. Have your gynecologist work with you to find the right oral contraceptive." She set up a Pulmonary Function Tests (PFT's) and stated, when another pneumothorax shows up, we can then take a look. She never accepted, nor bothered to look at the copied notes I made for her.

Today is my PFT's. Well, something has got to show. The technician wants me to 'give it my all' so I will not hold back. I did not hold back.

Uh oh, that was a mistake.

Seriously. Just like the stress test. I am not feeling very well. Here comes the hot burning pressure again. I am not going to agree to anymore tests. I can't keep doing this.

OMG. It's about 36 hours since the PFT. Those chest pains never went away. In fact, they got worse. The Trans Siberian Orchestra just finished their concert (a tradition for us for the third year now). I can't walk. I can't breathe in the bitter cold air. I am crying. My husband and son don't understand. Every step I take, the knives are piercing my chest. My husband and son are on each side of me trying to carry me toward the car. I can't move my arms from the pressure they are applying to my chest to try to stop the pains. I just want to die.

I need to breathe. I can't breathe. The pain.

Extensive pleurisy of both chest cavities. Everywhere. No prescription medications controlled the pain. Trial Neurontin titrated over time to a maximum daily dose only caused me to fall over in the middle of the night on my journeys to the bathroom. When the memory gaps because a safety concern, after driving to pick my son up from school unable to recall how I got there, I discontinued using it. Two months passed before I could adventure outside the home for extensive time. Unfortunately, despite resolution of the large 'pleurisy' concerns, the focal areas of pleurisy that plagued me for years and years associated with menstrual cycles continued.

It's my first visit with another Gynecologist. The first Gynecologist thought I was hysterical when I went back to her after my ultrasound. I even had my husband come with me. I told her all of the crazy things that were happening. She said they could not possibly be related. From her body language and tone of voice I got the impression she was behind schedule and was not ready to deal with any complicated patients. She advised waiting another six months with a second comparative ultrasound. I told her the cyst was gone. She refused to believe me. Perhaps she did not want to deviate from her original plan of care. That would require more documentation time to report new concerns and establish an alternate care plan.

I told her I was scared to have any more periods and that I wanted OCP. I went on to explain the correlation of my symptoms and past history. Her first reaction was 'That can't happen', 'It can't travel that far'. My husband sat there, mute in the corner. I was angry at him for not coming to my rescue!

I grabbed her prescription for OCP and as I passed through the door. Turning, I said 'my general practitioner has referred me to a thoracic surgeon and sees the relationship'. Her eyes got REAL BIG, her tone of voice softened and she replied. 'Oh, please let me know what they think. She can reach out to talk with me'. The news ticker scrolling across my thoughts flashed out: I won't be coming back to you, thank you very much.

So here I am, scared. Waiting in the examination room of another Gynecologist. I'm crying! I don't cry. I'm a tomboy, I'm a fighter.

This second gynecologist is more compassionate. The physician and his nurse acknowledged my concerns and nodded their heads in acknowledgement when I discussed the wax and wane of my symptoms around my menstrual cycles and history of pneumothoraxes which were (Catamenial).

The gynecologist mentioned treatment of two women during his 25 plus years but their cases were treated with hysterectomy and both ovaries removed. I was so exhausted and felt nauseated after examination that included abdominal palpations and a brief internal pelvic exam. He was more gently, methodical and smooth in how he applied and released pressure while moving from point to point. (Note: as a Physical Therapist, the characteristics in a hands-on evaluation are important to me. I believe it 'tells me' a lot about how thoroughly they know the didactic information and ease at which this information is transmitted through the use of their hands.) As for his prior experience with Catamenial Pneumothorax (CP), I didn't enquire any further into the history and outcomes of both women. I am afraid to run. The pain. The fatigue.

...fast forward...

It's been eight months. Eight months of oral contraceptives that made me bleed, non-stop. For eight months I felt like I was oozing and weeping inside. Literally. It became harder and harder to move. Everything inside was sticking together. I felt like I was wearing a bodysuit many sizes too small for me.

I was offered Lupron and was told 'if it stops your symptoms, its endometriosis'. I was never told any side effects about the drug except 'hot flashes'. I did my own homework. My biggest fear? The escalation of symptoms a few weeks after injection that occurs before symptoms are supposed to reduce.

Uh, first, THAT scared the hell out of me! I could NOT handle pain any higher than it is. Second, not knowing who will develop some of the long-term side effects, like bone density loss, memory impairment etc. seemed to be 'Russian roulette'.

Visit after visit, over eight months, I entered the clinic. The more months passed, the more bent over and slower I walked due to pain every step I took, or position I sat and layed in. Pain I later learned, was from the dense adhesions that formed between my diaphragm, liver, ribs, abdominal wall, small and large intestines. Who knew what was going on in my chest cavity.

Little did I know, the gynecologist underestimated the degree of my case. Nor was he abreast of advanced interventions for the disease. Although compassionate, his didactic, clinical and theoretical approach to address my needs were insufficient. After a long delay he performed an exploratory laparoscopy. I awoke to a nurse "no wonder you were in so much pain. You are going to feel so much better."

My husband was brought back to the recovery area, his eyes as wide as dinner plates. The gyn arrived. He seemed a bit nervous and talked quickly. The gyn's body language at post-operative consultation revealed everything. I cannot hold grievance. I am angry at the dismissal, misdiagnosis, and numerous delays that, despite my attempt to articulate the progressive serious pain I was experiencing over the years, its empowerment over my career, ability to care for my family and even daily function for daily life, was met with misogyny, ignorance and lack of accountability on the part of those I trusted to care for me.

The ONE thing that changed my life from this point forward, a multidisciplinary surgical team who are dedicated to those with endometriosis – anywhere that is accessible in the human body.

I see women run. My 'opioid' for life, I relinquished from pain. I miss running, in my heart and in my head. My body can no longer endure the pain. The fatigue limits me to walking the dog short distances.

Watching the game show 'Jeopardy' has become our evening 'date time'. It helps me keep some focus and critical thinking ability. I couldn't think fast enough to answer the questions but it was something we did together. These past few years, some days are difficult to even complete a daily easy crossword or word search puzzle. The fatigue. The brain fog. The pain. It never ends.

…fast forward ten months…

Here we are. I tolerated the direct flight from Seattle to Atlanta. I have always loved to fly. But over the past few years it's become more and more difficult to tolerate altitude descents and ascents. The sensation of sharp daggers, gurgling and feeling of my lung pushing and pulling against the chest wall like a flag flapping in the wind has become unpredictable and intolerable at times. It's a sensation I have rarely described to people, especially doctors. The facial expressions after I have told them is enough to keep it to myself now.

To be honest, I didn't think I could walk to all of my pre-operative appointments the day before surgery. Having a nap in the middle of the day made it possible. Etched in my mind forever: when I met the gynecological surgeon that would lead the team of surgeons for my case, I stopped at the entrance to his personal office. I looked down at the transition between carpets at the doorway threshold. Without forethought, the reality was very clear. Crossing the doorway is the start of something new. It leads me to the captain of a medical team known for care, compassion and support which I have never encountered before. Not aware of it at this time but, even years from now I will look down when crossing over thresholds, that will bring me back to this moment in time.

It's the morning of surgery. I'm lying here in the pre-op holding area. I'm not scared of surgery. In fact, I'm numb. My only fear; despite the photographs from my previous exploratory laparoscopy last year that showed evidence of advanced disease and my long history of catamenial chest pain and pneumothoraxes, years of dismissal that my concerns weren't that bad, I'm still afraid it's 'all in my head'.

Numb, in limbo. So exhausted, I don't know if I can fight any longer. What if this team of surgeons are unable to help me? Honestly, if something serious occurs during surgery, it would be okay for God to take me. It's not my preferred outcome but if it is His calling, I am ready.

Things are becoming clear. It's Monday, five days since surgery. I can remember bits and pieces after surgery, but I do not recall much about the intensive care unit and transfer to me room. I love my nurses and have no complaints. My husband has been amazing! For someone who is uncomfortable in hospitals he has been fantastic! He assists with all my 'accessories' to help me get on my feet. He helps manage the catheter bag, IV lines, chest tube drainage compartment and epidural medicine distribution box AND, help me steer the rolling walker straight since the sensation in my legs is a bit 'off' with the epidural analgesia working.

There is nothing more powerful than a drastic event, such as a medical ailment and the journey getting to the other side of it, that tests a relationship and reveal the depth of love between two people. I am blessed to have a husband with such commitment and depth of concern for me. The journey of this disease has been pure hell, but the experience of this surgical event and his unselfish care for me has truly strengthened the bond between us.

Surgery was eight days ago. It would be my luck. The slowed drainage is great news. However, the persistent air leak, well, it's still persistent. I know what that means. The harder fact, the epidural that has been wonderful to aide pain management was removed yesterday. An epidural is limited to seven days post-operative. Removing the epidural has made pain management a lot more difficult the past 24 hrs. A sense of dread is creeping into my brain.

F*ck. It figures.

I would be the 'infrequent' patient with a lung that won't stop leaking following surgery. This is not a common occurrence and the surgical procedures, the integrity of tissues and each person's body differ. In my case, triple wedge resections (one on the upper lobe and two on the lower lobe), chest wall lining (parietal pleura) was removed and the outer lung surface was abraded to promote adhesion of the lung to the chest wall as preventive measure to reduce pneumothorax recurrence and diaphragm work on the right and left sides were completed.

I've interacted with others who have underwent a procedure called: Talc Poudrage. It is a form of chemical pleurodesis. A slurry of talc is administered through the chest tube (in my case, a 28french – 28mm wide tube). The tube is clamped shut. When the mixture enters the chest cavity, the party starts. Seriously, it's not a party.

It's over. The talc pleurodesis was effective. (It took 10 months after the procedure before I was able to speak about it without my voice quivering and tears streak my cheeks.) A necessary evil. (looking back at the event, while I write this story for the FemTruth compilation of stories, I am watching Kilaeua, the volcano on the big island of Hawaii, spew molten lava and sulfuric gas from fissures in the ground.) I recall my husband squeezed my hand. My eyes wide open. I can't speak.

The sensation was hot, suffocating and, at that moment, I seriously wanted to die. My nurses came quickly to my rescue with IV medication. It was enough to take the 'edge off', make me drowsy enough to lay there and 'let it be'. I understood later why the doctor was frustrated that the leak had not stopped. I understood why his Nurse Practitioner left very quickly after administering the procedure. I understood why the nurses entered STAT after the procedure was complete.

I got up late that evening to begin walking again. I felt so defeated but couldn't hold thoughts long enough to dwell on it. It was like starting rehab over again, only now I no longer had the epidural. The chest tube was still. The talc created a feeling of suffocation with hot pressure through one half of my chest. I had diligently gotten my lung volume over 1500ml before the pleurodesis (the item you inhale through a tube to make the yellow ball float in the container). Now I could only get the yellow ball to rise to a very painful 500ml. I didn't want to breath.

Although the talc chemical pleurodesis performed eight days after surgery significantly set my progress for activity the first weeks following, and seemed like starting over again, the reality was that I could not be discharged and begin preparations for journey home unless the persistent air leak was closed. My body wasn't going to do it for me, this was the least invasive way to close the leak. At least now I could board a plane and fly across country back home. If I was to ever undergo that procedure again, to address unresolved issues in my other chest cavity, I will hope and pray the circumstances will differ and it would be completed under general anesthesia.

I also realize that this entire process, leaving home for surgery afar, being helpless and reliant on my husband and those around us, has brought me closer to my soulmate than ever. The 'substance' and direction of our relationship feels cemented and more intimately entwined. It may seem corny but, 'to have and to hold, from this day forward, for better or worse, till death do we part'. Yes. This is how it will be.

…fast forward eight months…

I'm still in the process of recovery. The fatigue is improving. The brain fog is lifting. Continuous aquatic therapy and physical therapy is improving my ability to move, tolerate a larger variety of positions and eat a bit more at meal time. The adhesions had really constricted by digestive system to function properly before. I gradually gained the volume of air I could breath in to fully expand my lungs. I would like to return to my profession.

My severe deconditioning and slowed processing speed and tolerance to environments with lots of sensory stimulation is now a major consideration to where I can go professionally, moving forward. I recently completed my first three-day Women's Health Pelvic Floor Physical Therapy training course. Although I have 'dabbled' in a variety of areas: orthopedics, geriatrics, neurological disorders (spinal cord injuries, traumatic brain injuries, young strokes and post-resected brain tumors). My best love has always been balance and vestibular (inner ear) dysfunctions. Between my current physical capacities and tolerance for clinical environments that are commonly high physical demand and quick pace that requires an ability to shift focus often and repetitively through the day I needed to start easing my way back to the profession.

The first step was this pelvic therapy course. Attendance gave me an opportunity to understand and apply more knowledge to other women in the support groups, expand my knowledge base of endometriosis as an advocate and build my continuing education credits as a medical practitioner. It's opportunity for exposure into an alternate clinical area I could pursue, IF. If my body becomes more resilient and consistent to tolerate the rigors of clinical practice again. The course was fantastic. The hands-on learning experience was excellent. It was a good place to be. Most of the participating Physical Therapists were also new to Women's Health or have limited experience. Although I've been removed from clinical practice the past few years due to illness, I didn't feel isolated. In fact, when it came to the didactic information about endometriosis, I was able to offer updated, accurate information for them to consider for future coursework. The experience was exhausting but very rewarding.

There was ONE surprise. I experienced something I had never imagined. On the course's second day, the instructor opened conversation about the incidence of medical providers dismissal of women's health complaints and impact on the woman. The instructor then proceeded to play an audio account of a women who sought help for severe pelvic pain and her journey for answers. I had no idea of the emotions I had stored away. I thought I had closure. Many months of counselling. I thought I had worked through my feelings of the injustices by others that had taken so much from my life. The tears flowed…and flowed…and flowed.

Without even a visual memory being recalled, the emotions unleashed like a breached dam. I stepped into the hall. I could still hear the audio replay of the woman's account. I was covered in sweat, my heart dancing, thoughts swirling. I thought the only way I could keep control was to pace the hall. The reality of Post Traumatic Stress Disorder (PTSD). Never, ever had I felt this out-of-control. Never have I acted in this way in public. I was ashamed, embarrassed. But, when I re-entered the room, it was then, that I realized, I am among like-minded persons in a professional field that is blessed with opportunity to establish relationships with our clients. A trust that differs from other healthcare professions.

After regaining my composure, I found many of my peers in attendance who wanted to hear my stories and found significant value from witnessing my reaction to another woman's story, with the reality that it happens to our peer professionals within the healthcare system itself.

…a comment about gaslighting of persons seeking medical help…

As a Physical Therapist, I have never once, dismissed a person's complaints as false, made-up or imagined. Yes, we encounter persons who have 'malingered'. These persons often have original issues that are addressed through physical therapy services but a person may 'amplify' or 'lengthen' the duration of an injury or dysfunction for other incentives (longer period off work, financial reimbursement injury claim etc). But this is very infrequent and associated with other areas of the body.

Over the years as a practitioner, and my own personal health experience, the vast majority of persons seek help when they have a problem. Most people have a genuine health problem when they seek medical help. I also understand that each person's interpretation of their sensory experiences differ. It is important that their descriptions are not judged prematurely. I more often find that complaints that are not resolved for a specific diagnosis, are often due to an incorrect diagnosis and failure to identify other contributing conditions.

It is far quicker and easier for us, as medical providers, to dismiss a patient as 'uncooperative', 'noncompliant', 'drug seeking', 'malingerer', 'psychosomatic' when they do not get better with our care. It is a duty of all practitioners to first consider that the failure to improve may be due to our own insufficiencies or limitations of our own skill set. We should remain humble, express to our patients that we do not know everything. Instead of dismissing our patients, we should be stating to them our limitations, uncertainties of what is causing the issues and how to address it. An offer to work alongside the patient to find answers, referring to others when it is appropriate.

…fast forward, working in advocacy and adjustment to 'the new norm'.

It's been three years since I found a physician and surgical team who validated my concerns and knew how to treat me. It required a 6,000 mile journey but the realization was simple. I could no longer live life, the state I was in. The most recent journey of the unknown and travel for proper care was a turning point in my life.

During the darkest years before surgery, my appreciation for the birds who came to my feeder and bees gathering nectar from my flowers filled my senses and brought joy to me. There were many days, rooted in my gravity eliminated chair, just 'being'. It was very hard to accept, yet I was too ill to make a fuss.

It was a battle during the worst days, particularly when I feared a lung collapse, to summon the energy to seek medical help. The fear of dismissal and exertion was far more overwhelming to me than remaining in my own bed, or gravity-eliminated chair where I could control the sensory load from the environment, avoid the large copays of an emergency room visit and save my spoons (energy).

The disease process has left residual impairments I have had to adjust to. The woman with boundless energy is now someone who must carefully ration her spoons. It's taken a few years to crawl out of the deep dark void I felt devoured by for the past few years. I don't have sensory overload as easily but when periods of fatigue return its more difficult. I feel like I can articulate my thoughts and feelings far easier but I have lost the ability to multitask and switch mental activities and focus quickly. The hardest part, regaining a sense of self. Self-esteem.

The journey of the unknown that waxed and waned for 30 years was finally revealed. It's so simple, looking back, to explain the unexplainable complaints. Even though I am a healthcare provider, I struggled with dismissal and gaslighting by numerous providers at different periods of time. This created self-doubt and sense that 'it can't be that bad. I just need to deal with it'. I had so much doubt, that the morning of my excision surgeon, despite all the photographs of my internal organs which showed the effects of disease, I was still scared they would find nothing.

Yep. Even visual confirmation of what had been happening inside my body for decades the doubt etched in my brain was still profound. Yet, nine days after surgery, I was released from the hospital. Eight weeks after that, I said goodbye to my abdominal binder and assistive devices for walking.

…what was I taught about endometriosis in Physical Therapy school?...

How much did I learn about endometriosis is Physical Therapy school? Two paragraphs in a textbook. I do recall many female patients referred to me over the years in practice who were referred back to their provider due to the strong association of their symptoms to their menstrual cycles. I was never privy to follow up of these cases to clarify what their true pain source(s) were.

It would seem that a medical education, coupled with the experience in our own body would be an asset when seeking care. I did not find this to work in my benefit. Not until I found my DO a few years ago, at the age of 45 yrs. Most often, when attempting to describe my symptoms and relation to my cycles I was dismissed as 'exaggerating', 'that's impossible', 'can't happen', 'you just need to stop being so anxious'.

Being told by so many providers that this disease is 'too rare' angered me. The fact that the disease was not recognized and I was not listened to over the years angered me. I spent my life working toward my academic and professional dreams, only to have the disease process escalate in mid-life, robbing me of time with my family, career and hobbies angers me.

I became involved in the online support community nearly six years ago. It has been amazing to watch the awareness of women around the globe come together, through accurate support and education groups. I researched everything I could find about endometriosis in general and also extra-pelvic disease. As a medical practitioner and 'atypical' presentation of endometriosis who was diagnosed for thirty years, I entered the community with a different perspective.

First, I wonder how 'atypical' from 'typical' my presentation truly was. As awareness grows to the body-wide locations of disease become recognized and treated, perhaps a shift in the classification of this disease will result.

Second, my personal experience and, perhaps a blessing, that I was never exposed to decades of literature that has classified endometriosis as a 'woman's reproductive, or gynecological disease' my personal perception of the disease, from origins through pathogenesis and systemic nature does not parallel tradition. I am frustrated to find so much conflicting statements about the disease. It seemed odd to me that the basis of treatment for this disease has not evolved over many decades.

Furthermore, these treatment approaches are based on a theory that I find too simple, and cannot be applied to the entire disease. Yet science continues to adhere primarily to this theory and limit exploration of many other valid theories. As an outlier all of my life, to find answers, there are times in science when we must deviate from the bell-shaped curve and look to outliers. Outliers are a resource. When a theory only supports the bell, and does not explain the outliers. Perhaps finding the explanation for the outliers can explain the bell.

Over a year after multidisciplinary surgery, I attended a global endometriosis conference with surgeons, allied health professionals and advocates. I attended to see the work being done, and where I may find a 'niche' among the endometriosis community in the drive for progress. My personal experience with this disease and investigative research and attendance to this gathering solidified my focus. Extrapelvic endometriosis.

What's that? First, 'pelvic endometriosis' is defined as disease of the reproductive organs and surrounding tissue. 'Extrapelvic endometriosis' refers to endometriosis implants found elsewhere in the body, including the gastrointestinal tract, urinary tract, pulmonary system, extremities, skin and central nervous system. (Extrapelvic endometriosis. Obstet Gynecol Clin North Am. Jubanyik KJ, Comite F. 1997;24(2):411-440).

The growth of our support and education groups of women, cis and transgender persons with signs and/or symptoms suggestive of extrapelvic disease, with our group focus on disease of the respiratory system (aka Thoracic Endometriosis Syndrome), with larger numbers of confirmed and persons with 'suspect' TES continues to grow. The prevalence of disease in these areas are still estimates. But the case can be made that its 'rarity' is due to lack of recognition, awareness and practitioners whom could recognize the disease multiple presentations, locations and different pathological processes that lead to catamenial pneumothoraxes, hemothoraxes and pleural effusions, hemoptysis and cyclical chest pain to comprehensively treat it.

Extrapelvic disease is under represented in professional conferences, research circles and both medical education, continuing education and to the general public. Disease of extrapelvic organs and their systems are traditionally a small portion of investigations. Less acknowledgement of disease through research and traditional belief that the disease is confined to the reproductive tissues and organs combined with very little medical school education, which is outdated, contributes to the perception that disease in these areas are 'rare'. However, the past few years, certain circles in the endometriosis community have expanded their interest in extrapelvic disease.

'Rare' has become a point of agitation with me. The fact that the governing body of Gyn in my country does not acknowledge extra-pelvic disease exists nor, established guidelines to treat it, ruffles my feathers. Hence, my commitment to raise awareness of its existence, prevalence and debunk myths and outdated information about disease outside of the reproductive system.

As my journey, evolved, I spun off of a closed support group to design a group with more focus on objective information from 'best' research, calling out incorrect information portrayed through the media and raising my voice to those with the authority to improve care for those with this disease. The FB closed support and education group formed. Its final transformation has become: Extrapelvic Endometriosis discussion and education group event.

The primary focus has traditionally been about thoracic endometriosis. However, I like to think of it as an 'island for misfit toys'.

The group has two pages evolving, each dedicated to certain areas of extrapelvic disease. Over the past year and a half, the attempt to represent extrapelvic disease generated a 'mascot'. Her name is Trish.

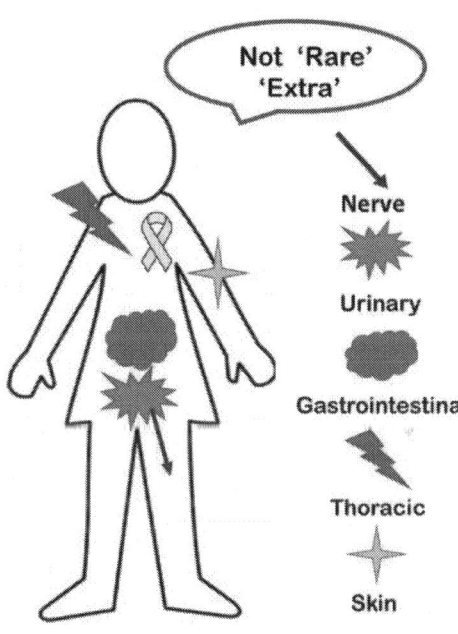

Trish helped provide a graphic representation of estimated extrepelvic disease subsets among those with endometriosis. Numerous visuals are available that state 1 in 10 women may have endometriosis. Trish provides a visual reference of the most common systems affected by extrapelvic disease.

A natural progression of advocacy endeavors led to development of a non-profit organization. (It's been eight months since the framework was created, and still waiting approval for licensure and 501 © 3 status). The non-profit is created with a specific focus: bring greater recognition of endometriosis as a systemic, body-wide illness that can affect multiple systems of the body.

Our goal is to educate providers and practitioners across the healthcare spectrum: emergency room, primary care and pediatrician, specialists and allied health for earlier recognition and appropriate referral sooner, not later.

Creation of a non-profit is far from my knowledge and experience as a Physical Therapist. I can verify it's not an easy task. Each state has their own requirements. At this time, the reality that my body is not reliable for return to clinical practice has placed me at this juncture. As someone who lived with disease for many decades, and the body areas involved, I was given an improved quality of life from my surgical team. They are amazing, but cannot cure aspects this disease has brought me.

I do manage a few residual symptoms in my other chest cavity (there is a significant preponderance of right sided chest disease. For myself, the left chest was more symptomatic and recurrent pneumothoraxes. The right chest is less symptomatic and without confirmed pneumothoraxes, hence I chose to defer this area). Given my age and other conditions, we (my excision surgeon) and I have treatment plan in place that is best for me. There are times my memory and bump from my daily routine can cause breakthrough concerns. However, these are a far cry from what I experienced before surgery with a multidisciplinary surgical team.

Here I am. Where? You may find me on the internet @ https://ExtrapelvicNotRare.org. You will also find Trish there. Please stop by and visit. It's a great place to direct your friends, persons whom may have endometriosis and, especially medical practitioners.

…I have shared snapshots through time of my life. But what was daily life like during the worst years?...

In my darkest days before surgery and the first year following excision surgery, it was exhausting to be around people, unpredictable events. Sights and sounds were overwhelming. Many days I was up long enough to drive my son to and from school otherwise I was in bed. Some days simple chores like loading the washer and dryer and cleaning the bathroom vanity ended with my in the fetal position on the floor from pain or exhaustion. I could not cook meals. I would burn them. It was exhausting to talk on the phone. I was limited in ability to sit upright to eat or work at the computer due to the pressure in my abdomen, shortness of breath and pain oscillating with my breathing. Word finding to talk was hard at times.

Somedays the pain was so unrelenting I would ace wrap my lower chest in attempt to reduce the repetitive ice picks when I tried to do things like peel potatoes or cut carrots. Many times my husband would find me lying over the ottoman with arms and legs supported on floor…trying to apply counterpressure to reduce the heartburn and 'vice grip' sensation running through my chest.

Some nights were awful. The only way I could sleep was to use bed wedges to prop my trunk up. Living in a two story home there were days where, when I was downstairs, I did not return upstairs until the end of the day. Even then, most days I had to rest halfway up the flight of stairs.

I had discontinued 'jogging' two years prior to excision surgery. Too many scary situations running alone on the paths. The chest pains and shortness of breath deterred me.

The disease progressed so quickly that many days I could not tolerate driving in a car more than 15-20 minutes. There were many times I had to pullover and open my car door, leaving my 'cookies' on the side of the road.

Adhesions seemed to advance so quickly that my rate of walking slowed immensely. Grocery shopping became my 'social outing'. I relied on the shopping cart to support my upper body. Meanwhile, each right footed step resulted in an uncontrolled 'grunt' and abdominal contractions from adhesions in my abdomen.

I even recall the night I rolled over in bed because the pain in my right shoulder, chest and abdomen was really high. Once I rolled onto my left side, I felt as if my body had been ripped in two. Well, not exactly. Lesions on my diaphragm had been 'oozing' for months (as the local gyns both convinced me that OCP would help control the disease process – even though no one had 'looked' to see what was occurring.) I told them that the OCP made things worse. I bleed nonstop for 8 months and felt like I was 'oozing; inside, everywhere. They assured me 'it's the disease process'.

Well, those lesions oozed, and oozed. A thick which adhesion between my right diaphragm and liver formed. The act of rolling onto my left side, with the help of wide pelvic bones, sleeping on a wedge, created enough lateral flexion for these adhesions to tear away. Not nice. In fact, I spoke to the local surgeon who finally did my exploratory surgery, exactly what happened and to look very very closely at this area. (!!!!)

The hardest realization for me, being the patient – I foresaw each step of descent into the providers view of the 'chronic pain patient'. It was horrible. The lack of energy, mushy brain from constant exhaustion and tolerance to stimulus plus the delayed rate of processing questions and conversations made it impossible to advocate for myself.

As a woman, I had encountered dismissal and gaslighting from time to time. However, the realization that women's health, and most particularly, endometriosis is a disease which is very misunderstood, under researched and healthcare providers are undereducated about all aspects of this disease. Most information taught is outdated and insufficient. With a prevalence rate higher than diabetes and asthma together, yet only receives 5% funding compared to diabetes, this is not acceptable. The more I learn about the disease, the numerous injustices, healthcare inadequacies and concerns for conflicting interest among the stakeholders of the endometriosis community, the greater my passion for change becomes.

Everyone admired my tenacity. Pursue and accomplish your life dreams. Fulfill your destiny. Despite all odds, I arrived at the destination I desired. My stay was short-lived. 'Life' had its own plans for me, whether I wanted them or not. Conquering, the unconquerable, drives me. Doing the impossible gives me 'self-worth'. Never the best at anything but I never give up. I'm headed toward a new destination, with like-minded advocates, may we get their together. May it be grand.

Submitted by Wendy Bingham, DPT   (February 17, 2019)

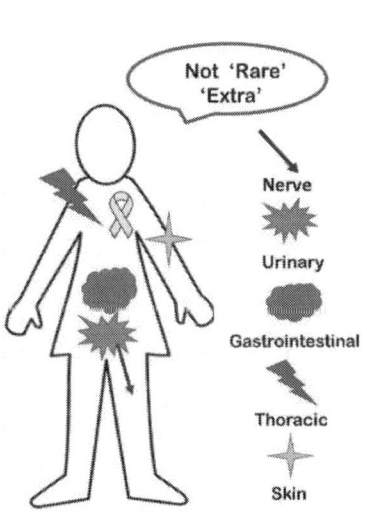
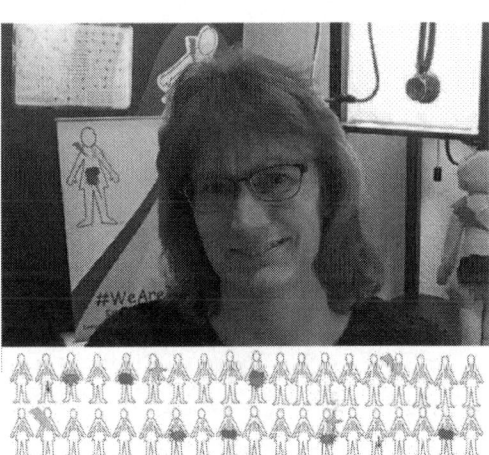
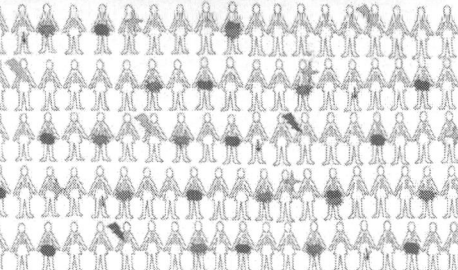

...."more and more, endometriosis is found in patients without typical clinical signs and symptoms..."

..."the clinical picture of endometriosis cannot be specific and widely heterogenous, with atypical signs and symptoms..."

"As a consequence, patients are frequently referred to other medical specialists than a gynecologist, with a frequent delay of several years before the correct diagnosis".

- Luca Santoro, MD et al.
Endometriosis and atherosclerosis: what we already know and what we have yet to discover.
Gynecology Ajog.org/article/S0002-9378(15)00391-p/pdf

Endometriosis Signs and Symptoms:
Typical: Dysmenorrhea, Dyspareunia, Recurrent Chronic Pelvic Pain, Infertility
Atypical: Gastrointestinal, Urinary, Respiratory, Cardiovascular, Neurological, Integumentary, Musculoskeletal

"Because extra-pelvic endometriosis is located in unusual sites, it is often confused with other pathologic conditions. This can lead to a difficult and challenging diagnosis and management. **In the presence of recurrent, cyclical and catamenial symptoms, extragenital endometriotic lesions should be suspected.**"

Yazdanian D et al. Frequently misdiagnosed extra-pelvic endometriosis lesions: case reports and review of the literature. J of Endometriosis and Pelvic Pain Disorder http://www.researchgate.net/publication/263673090

> "I'm talking, but no one's listening. I explain that my life isn't like theirs. It's not the same. And yet I'm labeled insane, but in whispers, when they think it won't hurt, but how can it not?
>
> I'm burning alive, from the inside out. Why would I lie?"
>
> – Silvia Young

TWENTY FOUR

Silvia Young, San Francisco Bay Area

How Does It Feel?

I'm standing alone in the middle, exposed, vulnerable, surrounded by everyone in my life that has come and gone. They claim they love me. They're all there, but they don't see me.

They see what they want to see when they want to see it.

But not me, only an essence of me, the part they need for their story. The superficial, super-sonic, super version, not me.

I'm talking, but no one's listening. I explain that my life isn't like theirs. It's not the same. And yet I'm labeled insane, but in whispers, when they think it won't hurt, but how can it not?

I'm burning alive, from the inside out. Why would I lie?

Why would you assume I lie. Why should I need to prove my experience. Do you live your life pleading with others for validation? What kind of patriarchy am I trapped in?

Alone in the center of the room, that's how I feel, encaged and enraged. Banging my head until I bleed, but it's fruitless. I learn to reign it in, I learn to act well, but it's draining my energy to pretend. The exhaustion of trying to fit inside your plain box, to ease your experience of me. It's a facade. There's nothing tangible for me to hold on to. If I let go what happens? I chance it.

Because how do you prove yourself when the system undermines your witness. When men and women take my words and twist them? An existence of non-stop pain misfiring and upsetting my game, drowning in gaslighting, financial assault without path for gain, there isn't anything endometriosis corruption doesn't touch. I'm left like a favorite doll, forgotten, not dead. but burning a whole bunch.

And no one cares. They want dolls to be pretty, fertile, and quiet. But quiet isn't an option because it's natural to scream when it burns. Self-preservation doesn't stop because you hold my safety net at a distance. It only makes me see you and your lack of worth to my existence. It shines on your ugly but how could anyone lack compassion, when someone says their truth believe them. You may be the last face, the last straw, are you holding the safety jacket staring at me, judging me. You do not know me, for my strength to rise despite your cruelty will bring my salvation, and you, you will still be coming short as a Human. When we think of our purpose, I know I reached mine. I know while my body falls apart, while my organs cement, while my psyche dances too close to the flame, that my heart sung truth, that I wrapped my arms around you and held my character as high as a rising balloon climbing above the limitless freedom of blue skies, higher and to its highest potential. I fly. And yet, I still burn.

That's how it feels.

I feel like an open book, I try to be in order to help others. My story is detailed in my memoir, *My FemTruth, Scandalous Survival Stories* (available on Amazon).

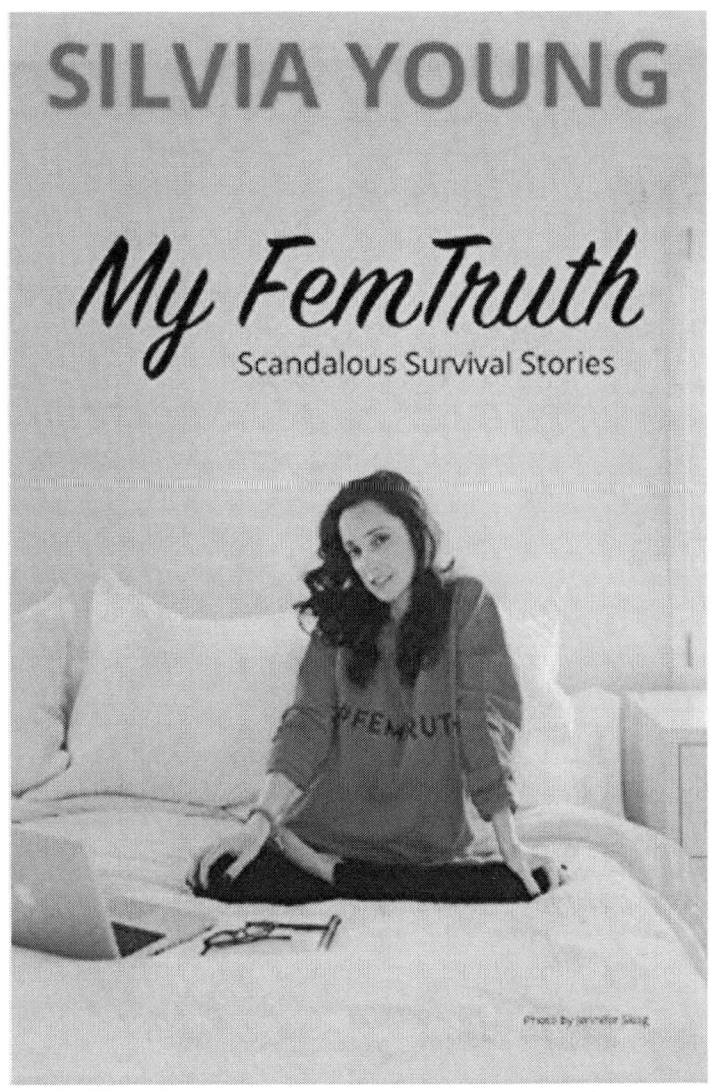

What you might not know is my behind-the-scenes work. This is my goal. This is what drives me. Until I achieve this, I cannot have peace. Here is the beginning of a policy proposal to help address the issues women suffering from endometriosis face.

Puff Legislation

By Silvia Young

In honor of "Puff" a pre-teen survivor and California resident. Stage 2 endometriosis ("bad periods" before menses) - EDS, POTS; pre-existing condition). Endometriosis is an example of a women's health epidemic ignored by current legislation, but only one of many).

To legally protect girls' and women's health and human rights by:

1) Providing accurate wellness education of women's health through all phases of life, including but not limited to nutrition and endocrine disruptors.

2) Holding companies targeting this demographic responsible, (liable/accountable for misleading/misinformation/nondisclosures) likewise, seeking transparency from all related agencies.

3) Providing diversability opportunities for the same quality of life beginning at 'I Believe Her', in line with the Schedule A (federal hiring practices and accommodations for disability).

Wellness Education:

Women's health, nutrition, endocrine disruptors through all phases of life.

Accountability and Transparency

Higher standards and regulations for companies targeting girls and women, and agencies charged with protecting them.

Equal Rights:

Access to non-harming products. Allowance and accommodations for wellness days with tools such as flex, telecommuting, technology advancements and innovation breakthroughs. To remove ableism obstacles to financial independence.

My fight is policy. Here I am am speaking at a rally about menstrual equity.

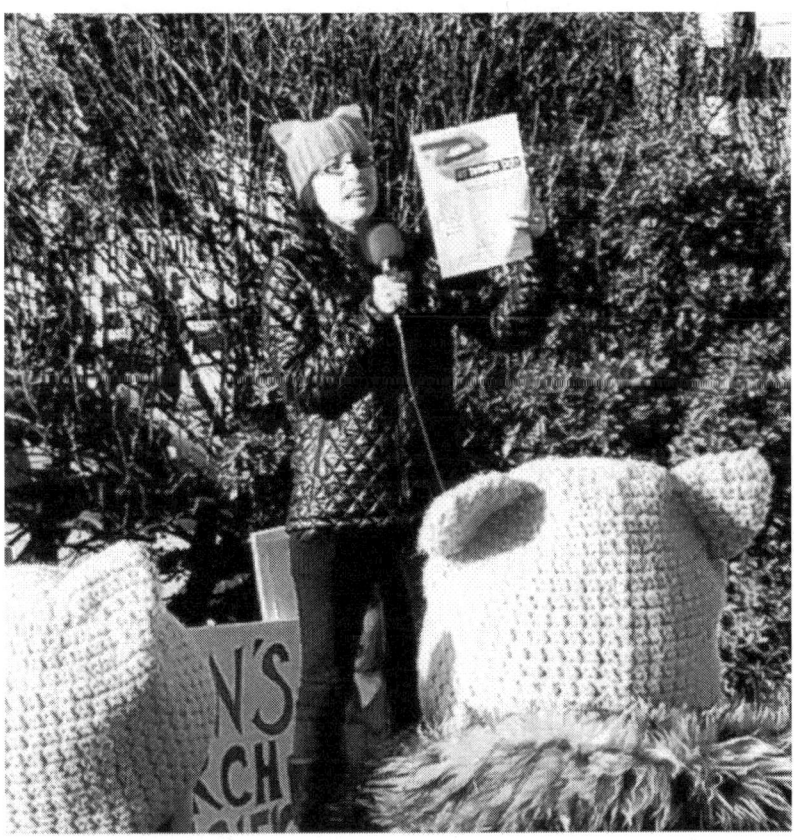

Alone in My EndoLife
- When I'm alone am I lonely -

I crave the solitude, the stillness of each moment not interrupted by my tired, tortured body. I feel myself pull away from everyday noise to be Alone With My Pain to contemplate this EndoLife and why it overflows with overcoming pure evil, struggle and strife.

Endo's history reads as cruel as any of the First Testament, I can't wrap my head around why the Womb was cast as the Antagonist, and the mob-mentality chanting "curse" instead of gratitude. Surrounded by the greedy intentioned magnifies my isolation. I can't break out of this hell - God knows I'm trying.

When I'm alone with my thoughts I wonder if this EndoLife is the total of me. It kills from within minute by minute. I try to crush it, rebel, but the enormity of it. One step forward, too many back. Patriarchy shackled me with EndoLife, spewing mythical fact.

I've been acting like I'm well, but now to act like I'm strong will be the performance of my lifetime. If you hear me singing, I won.

Thank you to the courageous women who shared
their endometriosis stories.

Believe them.

Our stories are our power.

Go now. Be empowered and share yours.

Made in the USA
San Bernardino, CA
03 December 2019